"This is an unprecedented book. Amen and F[...] prehensive textbook for all patients, which is [...] balanced."

> —*Thomas M. Brod, M.D., assistant clinical professor,*
> *Department of Psychiatry and Biobehavioral Science,*
> *David Geffen School of Medicine, UCLA*

"A must-read for all who struggle with these widespread emotional conditions, as well as their family members and friends. It should be required reading for psychotherapists and members of the general health-care field."

> —*David Grand, Ph.D.,*
> *author of* Emotional Healing at Warp Speed: The Power of EMDR

"Dr. Amen and Dr. Routh have put together a powerful resource for both clinicians and the general public to assist in the evaluation and treatment of the various subtypes of anxiety and depression."

> —*Mark Kosins, M.D., clinical professor of psychiatry and family medicine,*
> *Western University of Health Sciences,*
> *and assistant clinical professor of psychiatry, University of California, Irvine*

"This exciting reference will doubtless set a new standard for patients and providers."

> —*Dwaine McCallon, M.D., former senior physician,*
> *Buena Vista Correctional Facility, and*
> *past assistant medical director, Colorado Department of Corrections*

"An invaluable resource for physicians and those interested in establishing optimal mental health."

> —*Rick Lavine, M.D.,*
> *Practice of Psychiatry and Addiction Medicine, Mill Valley, California,*
> *and consultant to the American Dental Association*
> *and the Federal Aviation Administration*

"A quantum leap in the understanding and healing of anxiety and depression."

> —*Emmett E. Miller, M.D.*

"*Healing Anxiety and Depression* offers an enlightened view into these often devastating disorders, encouraging new developments in diagnosis and treatment in terms that can be appreciated by sufferers and clinicians alike."

> —*Samuel G. Benson, M.D., Ph.D., medical director,*
> *Registry Medical Group and Registry of Physician Specialists*

Healing Anxiety and Depression

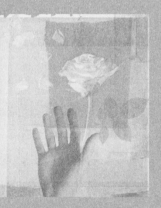

DANIEL G. AMEN, M.D.
LISA C. ROUTH, M.D.

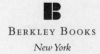

BERKLEY BOOKS

New York

THE BERKLEY PUBLISHING GROUP
Published by the Penguin Group
Penguin Group (USA) Inc.
375 Hudson Street, New York, New York 10014, USA
Penguin Group (Canada), 10 Alcorn Avenue, Toronto, Ontario M4V 3B2, Canada
(a division of Pearson Penguin Canada Inc.)
Penguin Books Ltd., 80 Strand, London WC2R 0RL, England
Penguin Group Ireland, 25 St. Stephen's Green, Dublin 2, Ireland (a division of Penguin Books Ltd.)
Penguin Group (Australia), 250 Camberwell Road, Camberwell, Victoria 3124, Australia
(a division of Pearson Australia Group Pty. Ltd.)
Penguin Books India Pvt. Ltd., 11 Community Centre, Panchsheel Park, New Delhi—110 017, India
Penguin Group (NZ), Cnr. Airborne and Rosedale Roads, Albany, Auckland 1310, New Zealand
(a division of Pearson New Zealand Ltd.)
Penguin Books (South Africa) (Pty.) Ltd., 24 Sturdee Avenue, Rosebank, Johannesburg 2196,
South Africa

Penguin Books Ltd., Registered Offices: 80 Strand, London WC2R 0RL, England

Every effort has been made to ensure that the information contained in this book is complete and accurate. However, neither the publisher nor the authors are engaged in rendering professional advice or services to the individual reader. The ideas and procedures, and suggestions contained in this book are not intended as a substitute for consulting with your physician. All matters regarding your health require medical supervision. Neither the authors nor the publisher shall be liable or responsible for any loss or damage allegedly arising from any information or suggestion in this book. The opinions expressed in this book represent the personal views of the authors and not of the publisher.

While the authors have made every effort to provide accurate telephone numbers and Internet addresses at the time of publication, neither the publisher nor the authors assume any responsibility for errors or for changes that occur after publication.

PRINTING HISTORY
G. P. Putnam's Sons hardcover edition / September 2003
Berkley trade paperback edition / December 2004
Berkley trade paperback ISBN: 978-0-425-19844-5

The Library of Congress has catalogued the G. P. Putnam's Sons hardcover edition as follows:

Amen, Daniel G.
Healing anxiety and depression / Daniel G. Amen, Lisa C. Routh.
p.   cm.
Includes bibliographical references and index.
ISBN 0-399-15036-6
1. Anxiety—Treatment.   2. Depression, Mental—Treatment.   3. Healing.   I. Routh, Lisa C.   II. Title.
RC531.A44   2003   2003043210
616.85'206—dc21

PRINTED IN THE UNITED STATES OF AMERICA
20 19 18 17 16 15

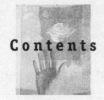

Contents

INTRODUCTION

ANXIETY AND DEPRESSION are major public health problems that are reaching epidemic levels in the United States. According to the National Institutes of Health (NIH) they affect 38 million Americans each year. Additionally, twice that number (75 million) will suffer from an anxiety or depressive illness during some point in their lives. The loss to our society from these illnesses is staggering in terms of individual pain, family strife, school and relationship failure, lost work productivity, and death. The Rand Corporation estimates that anxiety and depressive disorders cost the United States $80 billion annually, more than half of the nation's total mental health bill of $150 billion. Of the $80-billion figure, $24 billion occurs in lost workdays each year and more than $22 billion is lost from decreased productivity due to symptoms that sap energy, affect work habits, and cause problems with concentration, memory, and decision-making. Costs escalate still further if a worker's untreated anxiety and depressive disorder contribute to alcoholism or drug abuse. Still more costs result when an employee or colleague has a family member suffering from these illnesses. Anxiety or depression in a spouse or child can disrupt working hours, lead to days absent from work, affect concentration and morale, and decrease productivity.

Untreated anxiety and depression, more frequently than we allow ourselves to admit, rob people of their very lives through suicide and self-destructive behavior. Suicide, often the outcome of an untreated or ineffectively treated anxiety or depressive disorder, is the eighth leading cause of death in the United States. Sadly, suicide has tripled among teenagers since 1955 and has risen at an even greater rate among the elderly. Suicide affects spouses, parents, children, grandparents, friends, and coworkers, often for the rest of their lives.

Until recently, many people felt that anxiety and depression were the result of a weak will, bad character, or sin. Recent brain science has clearly revealed that these disorders are in large part the result of brain dysfunction.

Our work at the Amen Clinics has shed more light on the diagnosis and treatment of anxiety and depression by utilizing high-tech brain imaging studies. These studies have helped us to see the underlying brain problems associated with these disorders and have helped us target more effective treatment. We have learned that anxiety and depression may not represent separate entities, but rather a spectrum of disorders requiring carefully tailored treatment protocols for optimal outcome.

This book is about the exciting discoveries we have made and the treatment regimens we use.

CASSIE

As forty-three-year-old Cassie sat on the blue leather couch in the Amen Clinic, tears flowed down her cheeks as she said she could no longer focus on her work as the head of a nonprofit corporation. She could not escape feeling sad and nervous and being overwhelmed by negative, self-loathing thoughts. She said she was weeks behind on an important project and was on the verge of being fired from a job she had loved for more than ten years. The trigger to this episode of inner turmoil (she had had another period in college) was her failure to get pregnant. She had one child, an eight-year-old son, but was unable to get pregnant again, although she and her husband had been trying for six years. She always wanted to raise a daughter and was beginning to believe that it would never happen. She cried for hours every day and felt sad, hopeless, worthless, like less than a woman, and, at times, even suicidal. Additionally, she had frequent headaches, no interest in sex, and was very irritable with her son and husband. Her symptoms worsened during the last two weeks of her menstrual cycle. Her husband stayed at work longer to avoid her emotional storms. Her son felt the tension at home and had trouble focusing at school. She came to the Amen Clinic after she saw a story on television about our brain imaging work.

After taking her history and performing a noninvasive brain scan called SPECT (single photon emission computed tomography) we discovered that Cassie's emotional brain was dramatically overactive. She had too much activity in her limbic system, putting her at risk for depression; too much activity in her basal ganglia, causing her to feel anxious and emotionally stirred up; and too much activity in her anterior cingulate gyrus, causing her to get stuck on negative thoughts and behaviors. She had "brain reasons" for feeling so awful. To us, this pattern was very clear. She had Type 4, Overfocused Anxiety/Depression, one of seven new types of anxiety and depression that we have described based on our extensive brain imaging work. With the right combination of medication and therapy, Cassie began to heal. Because family members often suffer along with the person who has the illness, we included her husband in the treatment process. The brain scans helped her husband understand that his wife was suffering from something specific, not just acting badly. He became an active participant in her healing process because he wanted his wife back. As Cassie began to heal, her marriage strengthened, and she became a more consistent parent to her son. Cassie said the brain scans helped her better understand her illness, forgive herself for her erratic behavior, and be consistent with the treatment she needed.

Anxiety and Depression: Separate or Interrelated Illnesses?

Traditionally, psychiatry has diagnosed anxiety and depression based on symptom clusters rather than underlying brain dysfunction. However, ignoring brain function limits our diagnostic accuracy and ability to be successful in combating these illnesses. Based on the Amen Clinic's extensive brain imaging work, we have seen that there are at least five major highly interconnected brain circuits that underlie most anxiety and depressive disorders. Problems may arise in individual brain circuits or in a combination of them.

- The *basal ganglia* (deep brain structures) set the idling level for the body. When they are too active, people feel revved up, anxious, and on edge. When they are underactive, people feel slowed down and unmotivated.

- The *deep limbic system* (or emotional brain) sets the feeling tone of the mind. When it is overactive, people tend to feel depressed, negative, hopeless, and have appetite and sleep problems.

- The *anterior cingulate gyrus,* in the frontal lobes, helps the brain with cognitive flexibility and shifting attention. When it is overactive, people tend to get stuck on negative thoughts or behaviors (seen commonly in both anxiety and depression).

- The *temporal lobes* are involved with mood instability, temper control, and memory. When they fire erratically, people may have periods of panic or fear for no reason, they may have dark, evil thoughts, or they may be aggressive toward others or toward themselves (suicidal behavior).

- The *prefrontal cortex* is the brain's supervisor and helps with decision making, attention span, judgment, and impulse control. When underactive, people tend to have trouble focusing and often exhibit poor judgment. When it is overactive, people tend to worry and have trouble letting go of hurts and bad thoughts.

Understanding these brain circuits is critical for proper understanding and diagnosis of anxiety and depressive disorders. Until recently we had no way of looking at the brain function of individual patients. Through the advent of sophisticated imaging technology, the application of which we have helped pioneer at the Amen Clinics, we can see and evaluate which of these systems work well, work too hard, and/or do not work hard enough. Understanding the role these systems play in the genesis of anxiety and depression has led us to exciting new information in diagnosis and treatment and a new way of classifying these illnesses. Applying this technology while following the course of treatment and tracking changes in brain systems has led to more effective treatment. We do not have to rely exclusively on the patient's description of the problem, but rather we can address the underlying physiological issues and improve treatment outcome.

Brain Diagrams—Outside Surface

Top-down "outside" view

prefrontal cortex

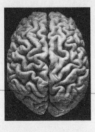

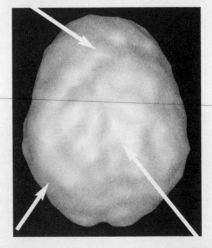

occipital lobe   parietal lobe

Brain Diagrams—Outside Surface

Underside "outside" view

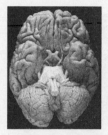

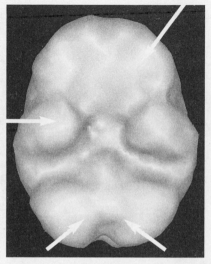

prefrontal cortex

temporal lobe

cerebellum

Left-side "outside" view

parietal lobe

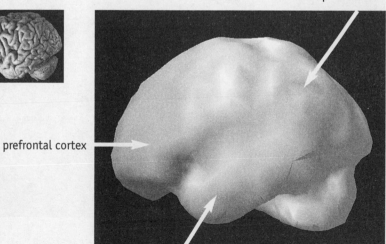

prefrontal cortex

temporal lobe

Brain Diagrams—Inside Surface

Underside "inside" surface view

anterior cingulate gyrus

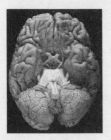

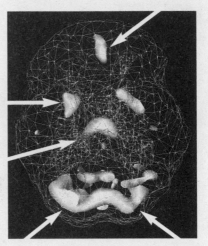

basal ganglia

deep limbic system

cerebellum

Left-side "inside" view

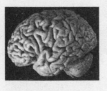

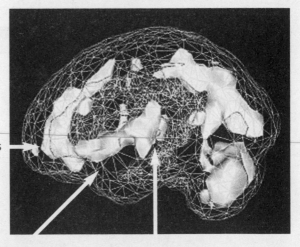

anterior cingulate gyrus

basal ganglia

deep limbic system

Physicians have come to recognize that anxiety and depressive disorders occur more commonly together than separately. When they appear together, they are associated with more severe symptoms, increased impairment, a more lasting course and poorer outcome, and a higher incidence of suicide. In one study, as many as 80 percent of patients with an anxiety disorder also had symptoms of depression. In another study, 70 percent of patients with depression also had significant anxiety complaints. There is also commonality between treatments. Antidepressants and cognitive therapy (therapy for one's thoughts) are commonly used to treat both depression and anxiety.

The Current Approach to Help

Unfortunately, most people with anxiety or depressive disorders remain untreated. A 2001 UCLA study showed that fewer than one-third of people suffering from anxiety and depression receive proper medical treatment. Although 83 percent of study participants reported that they had seen a health care provider for a medical condition within the previous year, only 30 percent had received adequate mental health care. Furthermore, only 19 percent of patients who had seen a primary care physician rather than a mental health specialist had received appropriate treatment for anxiety or depression. The treatment shortfalls were especially striking for African-Americans, the elderly, the young, and those with less than a high-school education.

The embarrassment, shame, and stigma associated with having a "mental illness" often prevent people from seeking help. Because we were unable to visualize brain problems, many people felt as though their behaviors and bad feelings were in some way the result of sin, a failure of will, a character flaw, or were simply made up. Understandably, then, they were ashamed of their problems and reluctant to seek help. When people with anxiety or depressive disorders are brave enough to seek help (typically from a primary care physician), most receive medication as the only intervention. The era of managed care has forced primary care physicians to treat illnesses for which they have less than adequate training. These well-meaning doctors often take a simplistic approach to anxiety and depression, assuming that one treatment fits all, which leads to many treatment failures. Usually, "medication only" treatment for these disorders is bad treatment.

While the right type of psychotherapy from a skilled therapist can be very helpful in alleviating the pain of anxiety and depression, knowing how to select the right type of psychotherapy and when to apply it can be confusing. It is estimated that there are hundreds of different kinds of psychotherapies, offered by a wide variety of clinicians, including psychiatrists, psychologists, marriage and family counselors, social workers, pastoral counselors, psychiatric nurse practitioners, hypnotherapists, and so on. Also, when patients with underlying brain problems engage in psychotherapy as the sole treatment for anxiety and depression, failure and frustration are common.

The treatment outcome improves if patients see a well-trained psychiatrist. Over the last fifteen years, a host of new medications has become available for effective treatment. Additionally, psychiatrists also know when to refer their patients to psychologists for effective psychotherapy so that they get the benefit of medication and therapy. Yet the high incidence of overlapping illnesses leads to many treatment failures, even when care is from well-trained psychiatrists. Many of the new patients we see at the Amen Clinics come to us taking two, three, four, or even five different medications, and they have seen a number of different psychiatrists and therapists.

A New Approach

A more sophisticated, comprehensive approach is necessary for treating anxiety and depression. The new approach needs to take the following into consideration:

- anxiety and depression commonly occur together;

- these illnesses are, in large part, the result of brain dysfunction;

- there are specific types of these illnesses; and

- there are a number of effective treatments that are specific to each type.

A major problem with the current approach to mental health treatment is that psychiatrists, and others treating mental disorders, never look at brain function. Psychiatrists are the only medical specialists who never look at the organ they treat. The lack of brain imaging has kept psychiatry behind medicine's other specialties, decreasing our effectiveness with patients and reinforcing mental illness stigma and noncompliance with needed treatment. Odds are if patients are having serious problems with their feelings (depression), thoughts (intrusive, frightening ones), or behavior (aggressive or self-destructive), the treating physician will not order a brain scan. He will prescribe psychotherapy or powerful combinations of medications without ever looking at how a specific patient's brain works. He will not know which areas of his patient's brain work well, which work too hard, or which do not work hard enough. This is the equivalent of orthopedic doctors setting broken bones without X rays, cardiologists diagnosing coronary artery blockages without doing angiograms or fast CT scans, or internists diagnosing pneumonia without ordering chest X rays or doing sputum cultures. Yet the state of the art in psychiatry is to not look at the organ it treats. Essentially, the diagnostic practices of psychiatrists have not changed for *150 years.* Because the right treatment optimizes brain function, giving a person more access to his or her own abilities, and the wrong treatment makes things worse and demoralizes patients and families, it is time to start looking at the brains of individual patients. Typing anxiety and depressive disorders based on brain dysfunction will be one of the next major movements in psychiatry. It will help us stop blaming difficult behavior on misguided will and lead us to consider and optimize the brain.

Typing Anxiety and Depression

At the Amen Clinics we have discovered that anxiety and depression are a diverse group of brain problems that require individualized prescriptions. The Amen Clinics have pioneered the use of brain imaging techniques in clinical practice, and we currently have the world's largest brain imaging database for psychiatric indications, totaling more than 17,000 scans. We see patients from all around the world. Physicians send us patients from Eastern Asia (China, Indonesia, Japan), Europe, South America, Russia, India, Africa, and the Middle East. Based on our research with thousands of patients using brain SPECT imaging (one of medicine's most sophisticated functional brain imaging studies), we have been able to see the major anxiety and depression centers in the brain. Our research shows that anxiety and depression are real, brain-based, and fall into seven different categories:

1. Pure Anxiety

2. Pure Depression

3. Mixed Anxiety and Depression

4. Overfocused Anxiety/Depression

5. Cyclic Anxiety/Depression

6. Temporal Lobe Anxiety/Depression

7. Unfocused Anxiety/Depression

Seeing the initial SPECT studies on our own patients dramatically changed our perceptions of mental illness. Looking at the brains of people who suffered from "emotional illnesses" helped us begin to understand the unique patterns underlying their illness and the tendency of these patterns to improve with treatment. We were, and continue to be, dumbfounded at the strong resistance by many physicians toward using brain imaging tools in clinical neurological and psychiatric practice to evaluate serious behavioral or emotional problems. Many physicians who resist progress and the use of technology say tendencies toward specific psychiatric illnesses in brain scans cannot be seen, the scans are overinterpreted, it is too soon to use brain imaging tools on patients (even though they have been available for more than a decade), and more research is needed before brain imaging can become a clinical tool.

Psychiatrists must look at the brain if we are to understand the problems we face. One of the criticisms of using brain imaging in clinical practice is that not enough published literature exists to verify its helpfulness. Yet there is a large volume of literature on brain imaging for behavioral problems. Psychiatric journals frequently feature imaging articles. Unfortunately, too few psychiatrists take the time to integrate the information. On our website, *www.brainplace.com,* you can see more than 500 abstracts on brain imaging for neuropsychiatric reasons. We should image the brain in people who struggle with thoughts, feelings, or behaviors because the brain is complex and needs to be better understood. We need more accurate diagnostic tools and more precise treatments specific to the areas of the brain involved in particular illnesses.

Many professionals have told us that our brain research and clinical work is on the cutting edge of brain science. We often respond that we have been "bleeding on the cutting edge" for many years. We have had many critics and cynics express their negative opinions of our work and the most vocal of them have never read our work or heard us lecture. It is natural for us to apply state-of-the-art brain imaging science to everyday practice because we search daily for new ways to improve our diagnostic and treatment skills for the betterment of our patients. Our patients' satisfaction and enhanced treatment outcome tell us it is the right thing to do.

To treat all anxiety and depressive disorders as though they are the same illness invites erratic treatment response and failure. In this book we:

- clearly delineate each type and show the underlying brain pathology (brain SPECT images) associated with it;

- associate each type with the current standard classification of anxiety and depressive illnesses. Currently, the Diagnostic and Statistical Manual of the American Psychiatric Association (DSM-IV) lists five anxiety disorders (Panic Disorder, Phobias, Posttraumatic Stress Disorder, Obsessive-Compulsive Disorder, and Generalized Anxiety Disorder) and five depressive disorders (Major Depressive Disorder, Dysthymia, Cyclothymia, Bipolar Disorder, and Premenstrual Dysphoric Disorder);

- give you a detailed questionnaire so that you can identify which type best fits you or those you love. The questionnaire was developed from our extensive database to *allow you to take advantage of our discoveries, even if you do not have access to the imaging technology in your local community;* and,

- describe a treatment protocol targeted for each type that we have found to be helpful in our clinics.

One of the unique features of this book is that a male and female physician team wrote it. Both of us are psychiatrists with special training in child and adolescent psychiatry and brain imaging, and together we have treated thousands of patients with anxiety and depression. Dr. Daniel Amen has pioneered the use of brain imaging in clinical psychiatric practice, while Dr. Lisa Routh has specialized in psychopharmacology, traumatic brain injury, and gender and hormonal issues.

This book is a practical guide to conquering anxiety and depression, based on new brain science. We are able to do this based on our extensive brain imaging database and clinical experience. In addition, we take an extensive look at *gender issues* in anxiety and depressive disorders. The incidence of anxiety and depressive disorders is equal in boys and girls, but as teens go through puberty, the incidence of these disorders rapidly escalates in females. We also discuss the *hormonal influences* on anxiety and depression, premenstrual tension syndrome, and postpartum and postmenopausal depression. Astonishing brain images of these states are included in this book, before and after treatment. By the end of the book, you will have an in-depth knowledge of anxiety and depressive disorders, the different types, and the underlying brain dysfunction associated with each and how to overcome them.

CHAPTER 1

Seeing Anxiety and Depression: Brain SPECT Imaging

Sean was one of the cutest, brightest ten-year-old boys with blond hair and big blue eyes we had ever seen. He came into our clinic clutching Dr. Amen's book *Change Your Brain, Change Your Life,* which his mother had given to him and which he had actually read from cover to cover. Based on what he had read in the book he predicted that he would have problems in his deep limbic system and left temporal lobe. When we asked him how he knew this, he said that he had periods of really bad depression, a very bad temper, and that he had tried to kill himself the year before when he was feeling really sad. He also said that sometimes he saw shadows and bugs crawling on walls when there were none. As part of Sean's evaluation we did a brain SPECT series. When we reviewed the scans with Sean it became clear that he had perfectly predicted his own SPECT results. He had excessive activity in the brain's emotional center (the deep limbic system) and decreased activity in the left temporal lobe. As he and his parents looked at the images on the computer screen, tears rolled down Sean's and his mother's cheeks. "I never wanted to feel bad or be so mad," he said. "I always wanted to be good. I guess I know why I had those problems." On the right treatment, guided by the scans, his history, and our clinical observations, Sean's mood and temper stabilized and he thrived in school and at home.

A picture can be invaluable. Once we started our imaging work we could clearly see that these diseases were in fact brain problems. From the first month performing scans, more than twelve years ago, imaging has changed the way we look at patients. Before we were able to perform brain scans, our approach to diagnosis and treatment was based on patient interviews and symptom checklists, such as those found in the DSM (Diagnostic and Statistical Manual) published by the American Psychiatric Association. The DSM, now in its fifth version, is considered by many to be the bible for diagnosing psychiatric illness. Unfortunately, psychiatric diagnoses in the DSM are still based on symptom clusters and have little or nothing to do with underlying brain dysfunction.

Shortly after starting the imaging work, we learned to use the scan images like radar to help us target treatment toward the specific brain regions that were abnormal. The greatest aspect of our work was observing that effective treatment causes a patient's brain to actually start healing. We could change brain patterns, see it on a follow-up scan, optimize brain function, and subsequently help people heal from the inside out.

Using brain imaging to help diagnose psychiatric illness was not part of our training, even though we trained at some of the most respected institutions in the country. Dr. Amen trained at the Walter Reed Army Medical Center in Washington, D.C., and Dr. Routh at the Mayo Clinic in Rochester, Minnesota, and Timberlawn Hospital in Dallas, Texas. Brain imaging is usually not a significant part of the curriculum in most psychiatric training programs. Although most psychiatric illnesses are strongly brain-based, psychiatrists don't look at brain function because:

- imaging is usually not a part of psychiatric training programs;

- imaging is not a part of psychiatric tradition;

- most psychiatrists do not know how to read brain scans or what the results mean;

- most psychiatrists are not sure how to use information from brain scans to help with diagnosis and guide treatment;

- many psychiatrists believe it is hard to get brain imaging studies approved by insurance companies in the age of managed care;

- most psychiatrists still perceive brain imaging tools as experimental;

- many psychiatrists are uncomfortable with technology.

We have argued for more than twelve years that it is crucial for psychiatrists to look at the brain on a day-to-day clinical basis. The field is changing, although much more slowly than we would like. We are actively involved in teaching the imaging techniques in this book to psychiatric residents and other physicians around the country.

Physicians have a number of different ways to look at the brain. MRI and CT scans are examples of anatomical studies. They tell us what the brain looks like, but not what it is doing and therefore are rarely helpful as diagnostic aids for neuropsychiatric and behavioral problems. Using a car engine analogy, the problem is usually with how the engine works, not how it looks. A car engine may look beautiful in a photograph, yet it may not start. Can you imagine how long a service center would remain in business if the mechanic's standard reply to a car owner's complaint was, "Well, it looks just fine"? Yet this is exactly what the vast majority of people who have brain dysfunction hear from the medical community after their EEG, MRI, or CT results come in. We have no doubt that in most cases these brains "look just fine" because the problem is not with "looks" but rather with how the brains work.

Currently, there are five ways to evaluate brain function:

Electroencephalogram (EEG), a technology that is seventy years old, uses electrodes to record electrical activity from the scalp and infer information about brain function. It has poor resolution and is rarely helpful for psychiatric purposes.

Quantitative EEG studies (QEEG) is a more sophisticated version of EEG that uses computers to enhance electrical signals, but still relies on inferring data about the brain through the scalp, skull, and coverings of the brain. Dr. Amen used QEEG before he switched to SPECT in 1991.

Positron emission tomography (PET) is a nuclear medicine study utilizing minute doses of radioisotopes to look at living brain blood flow and metabolism. PET studies provide elegant views of brain function, but the equipment tends to be available in research centers and cannot be accessed by large numbers of patients.

Single photon emission computed tomography (SPECT) is also a nuclear medicine study that evaluates cerebral blood flow. SPECT is the study we perform at the Amen Clinics. We find it the most practical and cost effective, and it provides amazing pictures of brain function.

Functional MRI, or fMRI, a newer study, is taking over much of the research in psychiatry. fMRI's advantages include no radiation, as opposed to PET and SPECT, but it is in the early stages of use with little clinical application to psychiatry at this point.

SPECT: A Window into Anxiety and Depression

Before we go further, it is important to understand SPECT technology. SPECT stands for single photon emission computer tomography. It is a sophisticated nuclear medicine study that allows us to visualize brain blood flow and metabolism. In this study, a radioactive isotope is attached to a substance (Ceretec) that is easily taken up by the cells in the brain. A small amount of this compound is injected into a patient's vein, travels through the bloodstream, and locks into brain cells. As the isotope breaks down it releases energy in the form of gamma rays. The gamma rays are like beacons of light that signal where the compound is in the brain. People do not have allergic reactions to SPECT studies. Special crystals in the SPECT "gamma" camera detect these beacons of light as the camera rotates around the patient's head for about fifteen minutes. About 10 million gamma rays strike the crystals during a typical scan, and a supercomputer then translates this information into sophisticated blood flow/metabolism maps and three-dimensional images of the brain. Physicians and researchers use these maps to identify patterns of brain activity that correlate to healthy brain function and those that are associated with psychiatric and neurological illnesses.

SPECT imaging belongs to a branch of medicine called nuclear medicine. Nuclear medicine studies measure the physiological functioning of the body. They are used to diagnose a multitude of medical conditions: heart disease, certain forms of infection, the spread of cancer, and bone and thyroid diseases. Brain SPECT studies help in the diagnosis of brain trauma, dementia, atypical or unresponsive mood disorders, strokes, seizures, the impact of drug abuse on brain function, complex forms of Attention Deficit Disorder, and atypical or aggressive behaviors.

Brain SPECT studies were initially used in the late 1960s and early to mid-1970s. CT and the more sophisticated MRI anatomical studies replaced SPECT studies in the late 1970s and 1980s. At the time, the resolution (image clarity) of those studies was superior to SPECT for seeing tumors, cysts, and blood clots. Yet, despite their clarity, CT scans and MRIs could offer images of only a static brain and its anatomy; they gave no information about the activity of a working brain. In the last decade it has become increasingly recognized that many neurological and psychiatric disorders are not disorders of the brain's anatomy, but are problems of brain function.

Two technological advancements have once again encouraged the use of SPECT studies. The early SPECT cameras were called single-headed cameras because they used only one imaging device and took as long as one hour to rotate around a person's brain. People had trouble holding still for that long, the images were fuzzy and hard to read (earning nuclear medicine the nickname "unclear medicine"), and they did not give much information about the activity levels of the deep brain structures. Then multi-headed cameras were developed with special filters that imaged the brain faster with enhanced resolution. Advancements in computer technology allowed for improved data acquisition. The brain SPECT studies of today, with their markedly improved resolution, can see deeper into the inner workings of the brain with far greater clarity.

We typically do two scans when we evaluate a patient's brain. We do a baseline scan during which the patient is asked to let his mind wander, and a concentration scan during which we challenge the brain with a computerized test that measures attention span and impulse control. We have found it most helpful to have both scans to see how the brain activates with or without concentration and to have a baseline scan for comparison.

We look for three things when we evaluate a SPECT study: areas of the brain that work well, areas of the brain that work too hard, and areas of the brain that do not work hard enough.

The images in this book represent two kinds of three-dimensional (3D) images of the brain. The first is a *3D surface image,* which captures the top 45 percent of brain activity. It shows blood flow of the brain's cortical, or outside, surface. These images are helpful for visualizing areas of healthy blood flow and activity as well as seeing areas with diminished perfusion and activity. They are helpful in looking at strokes, brain trauma, and the effects from drug abuse. A healthy 3D surface scan shows good, full, symmetrical activity across the brain's cortical surface on page 19.

The second type of SPECT images we look at are *3D active brain images* comparing average brain activity to the hottest 15 percent of activity. These images are helpful in visualizing overactive brain areas, as seen in active seizures, and many types of anxiety and depression, among other irregularities. A healthy 3D active scan shows increased activity, seen by the light color in the active scans below, in the back of the brain, the cerebellum, and visual, or occipital, cortex, and average activity everywhere else, shown by the background grid on page 20.

It is important to note that everyone's brain looks different. Brains are like faces and there is variation among them. From an aesthetic standpoint, on scans some brains are beautiful, while others are a bit misshapen and funny looking. Beautiful or not, from looking at more than 17,000 brain SPECT studies it is clear to us that a healthy brain shows good, full, even, symmetrical activity. A healthy brain has all of its major parts intact and they work together in a relatively harmonious fashion. While there are normal age variations, the brain scans of children and teenagers reveal more activity than the brain scans of adults; even an elderly brain, if properly cared for during life, looks full, symmetrical, and healthy.

When we first started studying anxiety and depression we thought we would discover evidence of brain patterns that would clearly define the two illnesses. We thought we would see signature patterns for each illness. We were wrong. There was not one brain pattern for anxiety and one for depression; there were many different patterns. Of course, once we thought through the problem it was foolish to think that one pattern would fit all people with depression or anxiety. After all, everyone who is anxious or depressed does not respond to the same medication or the same form of psychotherapy. As we studied the different patterns we made some other exciting discoveries. We noticed that certain brain patterns responded to specific treatments, while other brain patterns were made worse by traditional treatments. We started to use the scan information like radar to guide us in our treatment choices, and in doing so we saw our patients improve from the more precise treatment. Over time, we grouped the patterns for anxiety and depression into seven different categories and developed treatment protocols for each one.

Healthy 3D Surface Views

Top down

back

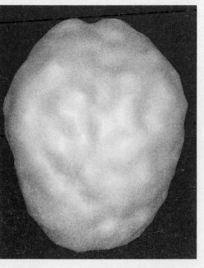

right   left

front

Underside

front

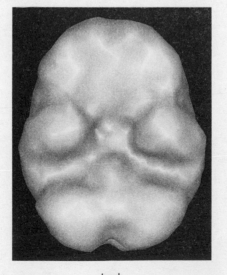

right   left

back

Healthy 3D Active Views

Top down

back

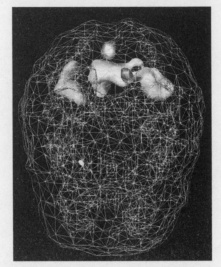

right   left

front

Underside

front

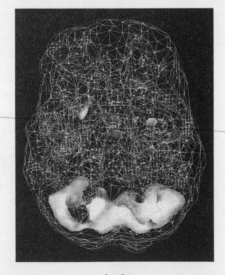

right   left

back

CHAPTER 2

The Brain Systems That Underlie Anxiety and Depression

The brain is the organ that ultimately experiences anxiety and depression because it is the organ of our personality. In fact, the brain controls mood, personality, intelligence, and adaptability. It experiences our hopes and dreams, sorrows and pain. Sometimes the brain is the sole cause of anxiety and depression; sometimes it is simply the organ that experiences the results of too much life stress. Usually anxiety and depressive illnesses are the result of a combination of brain vulnerability and life stresses. In order to understand the seven types of anxiety and depressive illnesses as fully as possible, it is important to understand the underlying brain systems involved in feelings and behavior.

The brain is involved in everything you do. The actual physical functioning of your brain heavily influences how well you get along with others, how you think, how you feel, and how you act. When your brain works right you tend to work right; when your brain doesn't work right it is very hard for you to be your best self. The brain is the most complex and powerful organ on earth. It is estimated that the brain contains 100 billion nerve cells, and each of these cells is connected to other cells through hundreds or, in some cases, thousands, of individual connections. It is estimated that the brain has more than 1,000,000,000,000,000 connections within it—more connections than there are stars in the universe. Each part of the brain is vastly interconnected with other parts of the brain. The brain is also very soft, about the consistency of soft butter. It is housed in a very hard skull with many bony ridges, which means it can easily be damaged. The adult human brain weighs about 3 pounds, or about 2 percent of the body's weight, yet it is the body's major energy consumer, using approximately 20 percent of the body's energy.

Although the brain is complex and interconnected, neuroscientists have learned that certain brain systems are specialized and involved in controlling certain functions. This chapter gives you a basic understanding of brain anatomy and the latest information on brain function as it applies to anxiety and depression. It is estimated that the brain has more than 2,000 individual structures. To make things more manageable and easier to understand, neuroscientists divide the brain into lobes, or larger systems. The brain is typically divided into cortical (outside surface of the brain) and subcortical (deep brain areas) structures. The cortex is divided into four lobes: the frontal lobes, temporal lobes, parietal lobes, and occipital lobes. A useful, broad generalization is that the back half of the brain takes in and perceives the world, while the front half of the brain integrates incoming information with past experience and plans and executes behavior.

Through our imaging work we have seen that there are five major systems involved with behavior. As much as we have discovered, it is clear to us that we are only at the very beginning stages of understanding brain function and behavior. The information we present here is based on our own experience and what we have learned through the study and application of what other scientists have discovered. What is thought to be true now is likely to be revised time and time again as neuroscientists continue to learn about the brain. The treatment protocols and diagnostic equipment that we consider state of the art today will seem primitive as technology continues to progress.

Basal Ganglia Functions

- sets the body's idle or anxiety level
- integrates feeling and movement
- shifts and smoothes fine-motor behavior
- suppresses unwanted motor behaviors
- enhances motivation

Problems Associated with the Basal Ganglia

- anxiety, nervousness
- panic attacks

- physical sensations of anxiety

- tendency to predict the worst

- conflict avoidance

- muscle tension

- tremors

- fine motor problems

- headaches

- low/excessive motivation

The basal ganglia are a set of large structures located near the center of the brain. They help integrate feelings, thoughts, and movement, which is why you jump when you're excited, tremble when you're nervous, freeze when you're scared, or get tongue-tied when embarrassed. The basal ganglia facilitate the integration of emotions, thoughts, and physical movement.

The Basal Ganglia—The Brain's Idle

Underside active view

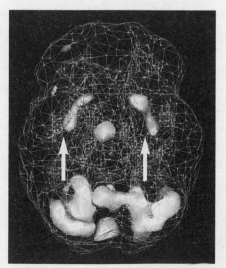

3D underside active view;
arrows point to basal ganglia area

They take in sensations from the body (emotions and thoughts), assist with putting feelings together with the correct body movements, and then help coordinate smooth outflow of motor (or body) movement. When they are working correctly, they keep input and output flowing smoothly, and emotions and body movements match each other. What happens when they don't work correctly? Panic disorder patients have basal ganglia that react correctly but to the wrong situations. Their basal ganglia incorrectly activate fight-or-flight body movements and a host of other body responses in response to the wrong sorts of emotional and environmental input. The fight-or-flight response is a primitive state that gets us ready to fight or flee when we are threatened or scared.

When a person has too much baseline tension or their idling level is set too high, we see too much activity in the basal ganglia and often chronic anxiety, tension, fear, and the tendency to have a negative or pessimistic outlook on life. Chronic states of anxiety and tension can increase the level of stress hormone production, and this in turn can lead to physical problems such as tension headaches, upset stomach, nausea, diarrhea, ulcer disease, and muscle soreness.

The basal ganglia have a range of optimal performance. You won't feel your best when they are performing above their optimal range or if they are underactive. People with underactive basal ganglia frequently have problems with energy, motivation, and decision making.

Of note, some of the most highly motivated individuals that we have scanned, such as CEOs of companies, have had significantly increased activity in their basal ganglia. One of our theories is that excessive basal ganglia activity may be associated with heightened anxiety or, alternatively, with increased motivation. If you do not use increased basal ganglia activity to get things done, you are more likely to feel anxiety and tension. Some people can harness this increased energy and channel it productively to become the "movers" in our society, but they may also suffer from strong inner turmoil.

The basal ganglia have been Dr. Amen's own personal motivator and nemesis. His basal ganglia are very overactive.

Dr. Amen: The increased activity in my basal ganglia has been both positive and negative. It obviously keeps me motivated and on the go, pushes me to strive harder to do better, but also sets me up for issues with anxiety and gives me trouble relaxing. Even though I wouldn't say I have a clinical disorder, such as Panic Disorder, I have struggled with low levels of anxiety my whole life. I used to bite

my fingernails, and sometimes still do when I feel anxious or it is the last quar-
ter of a Los Angeles Lakers play-off game. I used to have a terrible time speak-
ing in front of large groups, which I now love, thanks to putting into practice some
of the techniques in this book. My natural tendency is to avoid conflict or any sit-
uation that triggers anxiety. My mind can also play tricks on me and predict the
worst possible outcome to situations. Now I can laugh at myself when my mind
takes off on a negative course. For example, if one of my daughters was late com-
ing home from a date, my mind would see her raped, murdered, and her bloodied
body dumped alongside the road. Or if I narrowly avoided an accident on the
freeway, my mind played out the accident as if it had happened in great detail,
including the aftermath of paralysis, wheelchairs, and suffering on the burn unit
at the local hospital. My mind's natural tendency is to predict the worst, even
though I have been incredibly blessed in my life. Calming down my revved-up
basal ganglia has helped me deal with what life throws at me.

Dr. A's Anxiety Affected Brain

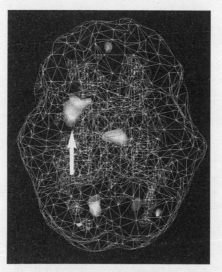

3D underside active view;
notice increased activity in right basal ganglia area (arrow)

Deep Limbic System Functions

- sets the emotional tone of the mind

- filters external events through internal states (emotional coloring)

- tags events as internally important

- stores highly charged emotional memories

- modulates motivation

- controls appetite and sleep cycles

- promotes bonding

- directly processes the sense of smell

- modulates libido

Problems Associated with the Deep Limbic System

- moodiness, irritability, clinical depression

- increased negative thinking

- negative perception of events

- decreased motivation

- flood of negative emotions

- appetite and sleep problems

- decreased or increased sexual responsiveness

- social isolation

The deep limbic system, called the emotional brain, lies near the center of the brain. Considering its size—about that of a walnut—it is packed with functions critical for human behavior and survival. This part of the brain helps to set a person's emotional tone. When the deep limbic system is less active, there is generally a positive, more hopeful state of mind. When it is heated up, or overactive, negativity can take over. The deep limbic system provides the filter through which you interpret the events of the day and tags or colors events depending on your emotional state of mind. When you

The Deep Limbic System—The Brain's Mood Center

Underside active view

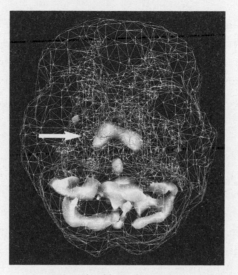

3D underside active view;
arrow points to deep limbic area

are sad (with an overactive deep limbic system) you are likely to interpret neutral events through a negative lens. When this part of the brain is "cool," or functions properly, a neutral or positive interpretation of events is more likely to occur. Emotional tagging of events is critical to survival. The valence, or charge, we give to certain events in our lives drives us to action (such as approaching a desired mate) or causes avoidance behavior (withdrawing from someone who has hurt you in the past).

The deep limbic system, along with the temporal lobes, is involved in storing highly charged emotional memories, both positive and negative. If you have been traumatized by a dramatic event, such as being in a car accident or watching your house burn down, or if you have been abused by a parent or spouse, the emotional component of the memory influences the deep limbic system of the brain. On the other hand, if you have won the lottery, graduated magna cum laude, or experienced your child's birth, those emotional memories influence this system as well. The total experience of our emotional memories is responsible, in part, for the emotional tone of our minds. The more stable, positive experiences we have had, the more positive we are likely to feel. Traumatic experiences in our lives increase our risk of becoming emotionally set in a negative way and make us more vulnerable to anxiety and depression.

The deep limbic system is also intimately involved in bonding and social connectedness. It influences how you connect with other people on a social level; your ability to do this successfully in turn influences your moods. When we are bonded to people in a positive way, we feel better about our lives and ourselves. This capacity to bond then plays a significant role in the tone and quality of our moods.

The deep limbic system, especially the hypothalamus at the base of the brain, is responsible for translating our emotional state into physical feelings of relaxation or tension. The front half of the hypothalamus sends calming signals to the body through the parasympathetic nervous system. The back half of the hypothalamus sends stimulating or fear signals to the body through the sympathetic nervous system. The back half of the hypothalamus, when stimulated, is responsible for the fight-or-flight response. This "hardwired response" happens immediately upon activation, such as seeing or experiencing an emotional or physical threat. The heart beats faster, breathing rate and blood pressure increase, the hands and feet become cooler to divert blood from the extremities to the big muscles (to fight or run away), and the pupils dilate (to see better). This "deep limbic" translation of emotion is powerful and immediate. It happens with overt physical threats as well as with more covert emotional threats. This part of the brain is intimately connected with the prefrontal cortex and seems to act as a switching station between running on emotion (the deep limbic system) and rational thought and problem solving with our cortex. When the limbic system is turned on, emotions tend to take over. When it is cooled down, more activation is possible in the cortex. Current research on depression indicates increased deep limbic system activity and shutdown in the prefrontal cortex, especially on the left side.

Do you know people who see every situation in a bad light? That actually can be a deep limbic system problem because, as mentioned, this system tends to set our emotional filter, and when it is working too hard the filter is colored with negativity. One person can walk away from an interaction that ten others would label positive, but which he or she considers negative. Because the deep limbic system affects motivation, people sometimes develop an "I don't care" attitude about life and work. They feel hopeless about the outcome, don't have the energy to care, and have little willpower to follow through with tasks.

Anterior Cingulate Gyrus Functions

- allows shifting of attention
- cognitive flexibility
- adaptability
- helps the mind move from idea to idea
- gives the ability to see options
- helps you "go with the flow"
- cooperation

Problems Associated with the Anterior Cingulate Gyrus

- worrying
- holds on to hurts from the past
- stuck on thoughts (obsessions)
- stuck on behaviors (compulsions)
- oppositional behavior
- argumentative
- uncooperative, automatic tendency to say no
- addictive behaviors (alcohol or drug abuse, eating disorders, chronic pain)
- cognitive inflexibility
- Obsessive-Compulsive Spectrum Disorders

Running lengthwise through the deep aspects of the frontal lobes is the anterior cingulate gyrus. It is a major switching area in the brain, with many fibers traveling through it to other destinations in the brain. We think of it

The Anterior Cingulate Gyrus—The Brain's Gear Shifter

Underside active view

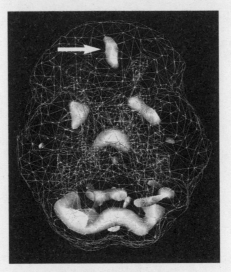

3D underside active view;
arrow points to anterior cingulate gyrus

as the brain's gear shifter, as grease for human behavior, allowing us to be flexible, adaptable, and to change as change is needed. It allows you to shift your attention from thing to thing, to move from idea to idea, and to see the options in your life. The term that best relates to this part of the brain is "cognitive flexibility." When there are problems in the anterior cingulate gyrus, usually caused by a lack of the neurotransmitter serotonin, people become unable to shift their attention and become rigid, overfocused, and cognitively inflexible.

Along with shifting attention, we have seen that cooperation is also influenced by this part of the brain. When the anterior cingulate gyrus works in an effective manner, it is easy to shift into cooperative modes of behavior. When there are anterior cingulate problems, people have difficulty shifting attention and get stuck in behavioral patterns that are ineffective. They are often uncooperative and difficult, or stuck in their own mind-set.

The anterior cingulate system has also been implicated in "future-oriented thinking," such as planning and goal setting. When this part of the brain works well, it is easier to plan and set reasonable goals. On the negative side, difficulties in this part of the brain can cause a person to see fear, predict negative events, and feel very unsafe in the world.

When the anterior cingulate system is abnormal, people have a tendency to get stuck on things, locked into things, to get the same thought in their heads over and over. They may become worriers and continually obsess. They may hold on to hurts or grudges from the past. They may also get stuck on negative behaviors or develop compulsions such as hand washing or excessively checking locks. One patient who had difficulties in this part of the brain said it was "like being on a rat's exercise wheel, where the thoughts just go over and over and over." Another patient said, "It's like having a reset button that is always on. Even though I don't want to have the thought anymore, it just keeps coming back."

The clinical problems associated with the anterior cingulate gyrus include Obsessive-Compulsive Disorder, eating disorders, addictive disorders, and Oppositional Defiant Disorder. These disorders are associated with problems in shifting attention. There are also a number of "subclinical patterns" associated with abnormalities in this part of the brain. The word

The Temporal Lobes—The Brain's Memory Manager

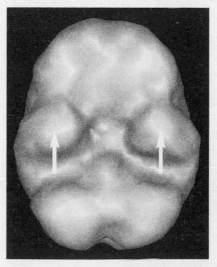

Temporal lobes (arrows)

"subclinical" refers to problem traits that do not reach the same level of intensity as a disorder but still cause difficulties in a person's life. Examples of these subclinical anterior cingulate gyrus problems include worrying, holding on to hurts from the past, cognitive inflexibility, automatically saying no, and being rigid.

Temporal Lobe Functions

- understanding and processing language
- memory formation
- auditory and visual learning
- retrieval of words and complex memories
- emotional stability
- temper control
- recognizing facial expressions
- decoding tone of voice
- processing rhythm and music
- religious experience

Problems Associated with the Temporal Lobes

- memory problems
- learning problems
- mood instability
- aggression, internally or externally driven
- dark or violent thoughts
- sensitivity to slights, mild paranoia
- word-finding problems
- unusual headaches or abdominal pain

- difficulty recognizing facial expressions

- difficulty decoding vocal intonation

- implicated in social skill struggles

- anxiety or fear for no particular reason

- abnormal sensory perceptions, visual or auditory distortions

- feelings of déjà vu (the feeling you have been somewhere before even though you never have) or jamais vu (not recognizing a place you have been before)

- religious or moral preoccupation

- seizures

The temporal lobes (underneath your temples and behind your eyes) are frequently forgotten in psychiatry and rarely talked about in clinical settings (outside of temporal lobe seizure disorders). Yet the temporal lobes are an amazing part of the brain, personality, and perhaps even religious experience. They are largely responsible for processing memories into long-term storage (damage here can cause amnesia), and they help you recognize the people you love along with those you'd like to forget. The temporal lobes have been labeled the "interpretative cortex" because, through an almond-shaped structure called the amygdala, they help you take in and integrate the current world based on your past experiences. The amygdala receives information from the senses, integrates it with past knowledge, and sends out signals for the body. When the amygdala fires appropriately, we tend to react to the world in a logical, thoughtful way. When it is overactive, we tend to be too reactive to the situations in our lives; and when it is underactive, we tend to act inappropriately.

The dominant temporal lobe (usually on the left side for most people) helps us understand and process language. It is also involved with memory formation and the retrieval of words. In our clinical experience, we have seen that the temporal lobes are involved with mood stability and temper control.

The nondominant temporal lobe (usually on the right side for most people) has been reported to be involved in reading facial expressions (getting the sense that someone is happy, sad, interested, or bored), reading vocal intonation or sounds ("It was the tone of your voice that made me mad"), and processing rhythm and music. It has also been implicated in visual learning, such as learning through seeing how things are done. In addition, the nondominant temporal lobe has been associated with religious experiences, such as flashes of religious intuition, and spiritual experiences, such as the one the apostle Paul had on the road to Damascus.

Temporal lobe problems have been associated with aggression, directed toward either others or the self (in suicidal thoughts or actions). One of the most important insights from our work has been the association of violence with left temporal lobe abnormalities, including dark, violent, or evil thoughts. Many of our patients who exhibit violence (murderers, arsonists, spousal abusers, rapists, bombers, and so on) have left temporal lobe abnormalities. We have also seen a correlation between temporal lobe problems and sensitivity to slights, mild paranoia, reading difficulties, and emotional instability. The temporal lobes have also been implicated in problems with facial recognition and social skill struggles. In addition, it is clear that temporal lobe problems have been seen in memory problems, and are the most consistent finding in amnesia and dementia. Unexplained headaches or abdominal pain are also common in temporal lobe abnormalities, as are periods of anxiety or fear for no particular reason. Abnormal sensory perceptions, visual or auditory distortions, feelings of déjà vu or jamais vu, religious or moral preoccupation, periods of excessive writing, and seizure problems have also been seen with problems in this part of the brain. The soul's religious experience (memory) and concern with God are likely housed in the temporal lobes.

Prefrontal Cortex Functions

- attention span
- perseverance
- judgment
- impulse control
- organization
- self-monitoring and supervision
- problem solving
- critical thinking

- forward thinking

- learning from experience

- ability to feel and express emotions

- influences the limbic system

- empathy

Problems Associated with the Prefrontal Cortex

- short attention span

- distractibility

- lack of perseverance

- impulse-control problems

- hyperactivity

The Prefrontal Cortex (PFC)— The Brain's Executive Center

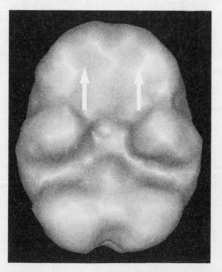

Underside surface view;
arrows point to prefrontal cortex

- chronic lateness, poor time management

- disorganization

- procrastination

- unavailability of emotions

- misperceptions

- poor judgment

- trouble learning from experience

- short-term memory problems

The prefrontal cortex (PFC) is intimately involved with executive functions, such as expressive language (clearly stating what's on your mind), planning, forethought, organization, judgment, and impulse control. The prefrontal cortex is the most evolved part of the brain and makes up nearly 30 percent of the human brain. Chimpanzees are our nearest primate cousins and yet the prefrontal cortex occupies only 11 percent of their brain. *The prefrontal cortex is responsible for human success.* It houses our ability to learn from mistakes, make plans, and correct our behavior over time to reach our goals. When the prefrontal cortex works properly, we are thoughtful, empathic, and able to express our feelings appropriately, as well as to be organized and goal directed.

The PFC helps you think about your words before you say them and about your impulses before you act on them. In social and work situations the PFC helps you review options based on your experience and select a course of action. For example, if you are having a disagreement with someone and you have good PFC function you are more likely to give a thoughtful response that helps resolve the situation. If you have poor PFC function you are more likely to do or say something that will make the situation worse. The PFC helps you problem-solve, anticipate potential consequences of your choices, and, through experience, choose the most helpful alternatives.

The PFC helps you concentrate by allowing you to focus on important information while filtering out less significant thoughts and sensations. Attention span is required for short-term memory and learning. The PFC, through its many connections within the brain, helps you keep on task and allows you to stay with a project until it is finished. The PFC actually sends quieting signals to the limbic (emotional) and sensory parts of the brain. When there is a need to focus, the PFC decreases the distracting input from other brain areas.

It helps to inhibit or filter out distractions. When the PFC is underactive, there is less of a filtering mechanism available and distractibility becomes a problem.

Thoughtfulness and impulse control are heavily influenced by the PFC. The ability to think through the consequences of behavior is essential to effective living. Good forethought is needed in choosing a good mate, interacting with customers, dealing with difficult children, spending money, and driving on the freeway. Without proper PFC function, it is difficult to act in consistently thoughtful ways and impulses take over.

The PFC has many connections to the limbic system, the emotional brain. It sends inhibitory messages that help keep emotions under control. It helps you "use your head along with your emotions." When there is damage or underactivity in this part of the brain, especially on the left side, the PFC cannot appropriately inhibit the limbic system. This leads to an increased vulnerability to depression. A classic example of this problem occurs in people who have had left frontal lobe strokes. Sixty percent of patients with these strokes develop a major depression within a year. The PFC is also the part of the brain that allows you to feel and express emotions—to feel happiness, sadness, joy, and love. The PFC translates the feelings of the limbic system (the emotional brain) into recognizable feelings, emotions, and words, such as love, passion, and hate. Underactivity or damage in this part of the brain often leads to a decreased ability to express thoughts and feelings.

When there are problems in the PFC, the organization of daily life becomes difficult and internal supervision (conscience) goes awry. Difficulty with impulse control often leads people with PFC problems to do things that they later regret.

We have based our anxiety/depression typology on single or combinations of abnormalities of each of these five systems together with the symptom clusters associated with each.

1. Pure Anxiety—based on excessive activity in the basal ganglia

2. Pure Depression—based on excessive activity in the deep limbic system

3. Mixed Anxiety and Depression—based on excessive activity in the basal ganglia and the deep limbic system

4. Overfocused Anxiety/Depression—based on excessive activity in the anterior cingulate gyrus, the basal ganglia, and/or the deep limbic system

5. Cyclic Anxiety/Depression—based on focal (a discrete area) increased activity in the deep limbic system and/or in the basal ganglia

6. Temporal Lobe Anxiety/Depression—based on increased or decreased activity in the temporal lobes and increased activity in the basal ganglia and/or deep limbic system

7. Unfocused Anxiety/Depression—based on decreased activity in the prefrontal cortex and increased activity in the basal ganglia and/or deep limbic system.

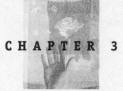

CHAPTER 3

Determining Your Type:
The Amen Clinic Anxiety/Depression
Type Questionnaire

The day-to-day use of functional brain imaging in clinical practice is, unfortunately, still five to ten years away. As we amassed a database of more than 17,000 brain SPECT studies and more than 12,000 patient evaluations, we saw patterns emerge. We identified seven different types of anxiety and depression that correlated with specific symptom clusters seen in our patients.

The Amen Clinic Anxiety/Depression Type Questionnaire is a 70-question self-administered test that screens for anxiety and depressive syndromes. Self-report questionnaires have advantages and limitations. They are quick, inexpensive, and easy to score. On the other hand, people may fill out questionnaires portraying themselves in a way they want to be perceived, resulting in self-report bias. For example, some people exaggerate their experience and mark all of the symptoms as a frequent problem, in essence saying, "I'm glad to have a problem so that I can get help, be sick, or have an excuse for the problems I have." Others are in total denial. They do not want to see any personal flaws, and they do not check any symptoms as problematic, in essence saying, "I'm OK. There's nothing wrong with me. Leave me alone."

Not all self-report bias is intentional. People may genuinely have difficulty expressing how they feel. Sometimes family members or friends are able to provide insight into a loved one's level of functioning, and they may have noticed things that the loved one hasn't.

If you choose to take the self-test, we believe that having another person fill out the questionnaire as well will give you a more accurate assessment. The person you choose to complete the questionnaire should know you well and be as unbiased as possible.

Questionnaires of any sort should never be used alone as an assessment tool. Like an isolated laboratory test result, they are not meant to provide a diagnosis. They are simply catalysts to initiate the process of seeking treatment. The Amen Clinic Anxiety/Depression Type Questionnaire is a valuable tool to help determine whether or not you or a loved one is suffering from one of the types of anxiety and/or depression. A person may have more than one type of anxiety and/or depression, and this underscores the need for a more complete assessment from a mental health provider.

The Amen Clinic Anxiety/Depression Type Questionnaire

Copyright 2003 Daniel Amen, M.D.; Lisa Routh, M.D.

Please rate yourself on each of the symptoms listed below using the following scale. If possible, to give us the most complete picture, have another person who knows you well (such as a spouse, lover, or parent) rate you as well. List other person _____

0	1	2	3	4	NA
Never	Rarely	Occasionally	Frequently	Very Frequently	Not Applicable/ Not Known

Other   Self

_____ _____ 1. Frequent feelings of nervousness or anxiety

_____ _____ 2. Panic attacks

_____ _____ 3. Avoidance of places because of fear of having an anxiety attack

_____ _____ 4. Symptoms of heightened muscle tension (headaches, sore muscles, hand tremors)

_____ _____ 5. Periods of heart pounding, nausea, or dizziness (not exercise related)

_____ _____ 6. Tendency to predict the worst

_____ _____ 7. Multiple, persistent fears or phobias (such as dying, doing something crazy)

_____ _____ 8. Conflict avoidance

_____ _____ 9. Excessive fear of being judged or scrutinized by others

_____ _____ 10. Easily startled or tendency to freeze in anxiety-provoking or intense situations

_____ _____ 11. Seemingly shy, timid, and easily embarrassed

_____ _____ 12. Bites fingernails or picks skin

_____ _____ 13. Persistent sad or "empty" mood

_____ _____ 14. Loss of interest in or pleasure from activities that are usually fun, including sex

_____ _____ 15. Restlessness, irritability, or excessive crying

_____ _____ 16. Feelings of guilt, worthlessness, helplessness, hopelessness, pessimism

_____ _____ 17. Sleeping too much or too little, early-morning awakening

_____ _____ 18. Appetite and/or weight loss, or overeating and weight gain

_____ _____ 19. Decreased energy, fatigue, feeling "slowed down"

_____ _____ 20. Thoughts of death or suicide, or suicide attempts

_____ _____ 21. Difficulty concentrating, remembering, or making decisions

_____ _____ 22. Persistent physical symptoms that do not respond to treatment, such as headaches, digestive disorders, and chronic pain

_____ _____ 23. Persistent negativity or chronic low self-esteem

_____ _____ 24. Persistent feeling of dissatisfaction or boredom

_____ _____ 25. Excessive or senseless worrying

_____ _____ 26. Upset when things are out of place or don't go the way you planned

_____ _____ 27. Tendency to be oppositional or argumentative

_____ _____ 28. Tendency to have repetitive negative or anxious thoughts

_____ _____ 29. Tendency toward compulsive behaviors

_____ _____ 30. Intense dislike of change

_____ _____ 31. Tendency to hold grudges

(continued)

_____ _____ 32. Difficulty seeing options in situations

_____ _____ 33. Tendency to hold on to own opinion and not listen to others

_____ _____ 34. Needing to have things done a certain way or you become very upset

_____ _____ 35. Others complain that you worry too much

_____ _____ 36. Tendency to say no without first thinking about question

_____ _____ 37. Periods of abnormally elevated, depressed, or anxious mood

_____ _____ 38. Periods of decreased need for sleep, feeling energetic on dramatically less sleep than usual

_____ _____ 39. Periods of grandiose notions

_____ _____ 40. Periods of increased talking or pressured speech

_____ _____ 41. Periods of too many thoughts racing through your mind

_____ _____ 42. Periods of markedly increased energy

_____ _____ 43. Periods of poor judgment that lead to risk-taking behavior (separate from usual behavior)

_____ _____ 44. Periods of inappropriate social behavior

_____ _____ 45. Periods of irritability or aggression

_____ _____ 46. Periods of delusional or psychotic thinking

_____ _____ 47. Short fuse or periods of extreme irritability

_____ _____ 48. Periods of rage with little provocation

_____ _____ 49. Often misinterprets comments as negative when they are not

_____ _____ 50. Periods of spaciness or confusion

_____ _____ 51. Periods of panic and/or fear for no specific reason

_____ _____ 52. Visual or auditory changes, such as seeing shadows or hearing muffled sounds

_____ _____ 53. Frequent periods of déjà vu (feeling of being somewhere you have never been)

_____ _____ 54. Sensitivity or mild paranoia

_____ _____ 55. Headaches or abdominal pain of uncertain origin

_____ _____ 56. History of a head injury or family history of violence or explosiveness

_____ _____ 57. Dark thoughts, may involve suicidal or homicidal thoughts

_____ _____ 58. Periods of forgetfulness or memory problems

_____ _____ 59. Trouble staying focused

_____ _____ 60. Spaciness or feeling in a fog

_____ _____ 61. Overwhelmed by tasks of daily living

_____ _____ 62. Feels tired, sluggish, or slow-moving

_____ _____ 63. Procrastination, failure to finish things

_____ _____ 64. Chronic boredom

_____ _____ 65. Loses things

_____ _____ 66. Easily distracted

_____ _____ 67. Forgetful

_____ _____ 68. Poor planning skills

_____ _____ 69. Difficulty expressing feelings

_____ _____ 70. Difficulty expressing empathy for others

The Amen Clinic Anxiety/Depression Type Questionnaire Scoring Key

For each of the groups listed below, add up the number of answers that were scored a 3 or 4 and note it in the space provided. A cutoff score is provided with each type. Some people score positively in more than one group; some score positively in three or four groups. Use the results to help guide you through the treatment sections of this book.

1. Pure Anxiety (Questions 1 through 12)

If you scored six or more questions with a 3 (frequently) or 4 (very frequently), you have met the criteria for Pure Anxiety. If you scored four or five questions with a 3 or 4, you have not met the criteria for Pure Anxiety, but you have significant anxiety symptoms.

Pure Anxiety score of 3 or 4: _____

2. Pure Depression (Questions 13 through 24)

If you scored six or more questions with a 3 (frequently) or 4 (very frequently), you have met the criteria for Pure Depression. If you scored four or five questions with a 3 or 4, you have not met the criteria for Pure Depression, but you have significant depression symptoms.

Pure Depression score of 3 or 4: _____

3. Mixed Anxiety and Depression (Questions 1 through 24)

If you scored six or more of questions 1 through 12 with a 3 (frequently) or 4 (very frequently) and six or more of questions 13 through 24 with a 3 or 4, you have met the criteria for Mixed Anxiety and Depression.

Mixed Anxiety and Depression score of 3 or 4: _____

4. Overfocused Anxiety/Depression (Questions 25 through 36)

Meets the criteria for Pure Anxiety and/or Depression and also scores six or more on the Overfocused Anxiety/Depression questions.

Overfocused Anxiety/Depression score of 3 or 4: _____

5. Cyclic Anxiety/Depression (Questions 37 through 46)

Meets the criteria for Pure Anxiety and/or Depression and also scores six or more on the Cyclic Anxiety/Depression questions.

Cyclic score of 3 or 4: _____

6. Temporal Lobe Anxiety/Depression (Questions 47 through 58)

Meets the criteria for Pure Anxiety and/or Depression and also scores six or more on the Temporal Lobe Anxiety/Depression questions.

Temporal Lobe score of 3 or 4: _____

7. Unfocused Anxiety/Depression (Questions 59 through 70)

Meets the criteria for Pure Anxiety and/or Depression and also scores six or more on the Prefrontal Cortex Anxiety/Depression questions.

Unfocused Anxiety/Depression score of 3 or 4: _____

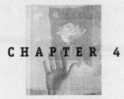

CHAPTER 4

The Seven Types

nxiety and depression are real illnesses. When left untreated they often have serious consequences and are responsible for school and job failure, relationship breakups, health problems, and sometimes suicide. We have discovered that these illnesses are not single disorders that occur separately, but rather are a cluster of closely related disorders. Understanding the specific type of anxiety and/or depression you have is critical to getting the most effective treatment.

The best way to understand each type of anxiety and depression is through real-life stories. In this chapter there are twenty-one short stories illustrating the seven types of anxiety and depression throughout the life cycle. These are actual case studies, real stories about people we have treated. The names and some of the details have been altered to protect the confidentiality of our patients. We have included a childhood, teen, and adult story for each type of anxiety and depression. After reading these vignettes, you will begin to see the complexity of anxiety and depression and identify the primary symptoms of each type and their impact on daily life. You will also note that in most stories there are family members who also have similar symptoms. Many of these problems have strong genetic underpinnings. This "life cycle approach" is very important, even for adult sufferers, because these disorders often begin in childhood or adolescence. Additionally, we list the major symptoms of each type and briefly describe treatments. (Treatments for each type will be more fully discussed in chapters 6 through 12.)

Type 1: Pure Anxiety

Pure Anxiety results from too much activity in the brain's basal ganglia. Sufferers feel stirred up, anxious, or nervous. They often feel uncomfortable in their own skin. They report feeling as though they "could climb the walls" or that they are "crawling out of their skin." They are plagued by feelings of panic, fear, and self-doubt, and suffer the physical feelings of anxiety as well, such as muscle tension, nail biting, headaches, abdominal pain, heart palpitations, shortness of breath, and sore muscles. It is as if they have an overload of tension and emotion. The symptoms may be a consistently disruptive presence or may come in unexpected waves. Irrational fears or phobias may also be a burden. People suffering from Pure Anxiety tend to avoid anything that makes them anxious or uncomfortable, such as places or people that might trigger panic attacks or interpersonal conflict. People with Pure Anxiety tend to predict the worst and look to the future with fear. They may be excessively shy or startle easily, or they may freeze in emotionally charged situations. Generalized Anxiety Disorder and phobias are examples of illnesses that fit into this category. The SPECT series finding of Type 1, Pure Anxiety is increased activity in the basal ganglia, seen on both the concentration and baseline studies. The twelve most common symptoms of Pure Anxiety are:

1. Frequent feelings of nervousness or anxiety

2. Panic attacks

3. Avoidance of places for fear of having an anxiety attack

4. Heightened muscle tension (headaches, sore muscles, hand tremors)

5. Periods of heart pounding, nausea, or dizziness

6. Tendency to predict the worst

7. Multiple, persistent fears or phobias (such as dying, doing something crazy)

8. Conflict avoidance

9. Excessive fear of being judged or scrutinized by others

10. Easily startled or tendency to freeze in anxiety-provoking or intense situations

11. Seemingly shy, timid, and easily embarrassed

12. Bites fingernails or picks skin

SAM

Waves of terror engulfed six-year-old Sam every time he saw a dog. The size of the dog didn't matter; little dogs and large dogs alike made Sam run away or cry out in fear. One day, Sam and his mother were out for a walk, holding hands and talking about his schoolday. Suddenly, Sam saw a small dog coming toward them. Panic-stricken, Sam jerked his hand free from his mother's and ran into the street to avoid the dog. While his mother chased Sam and watched in horror, a car swerved and barely missed hitting him. Terrified, his mother called our office to get Sam help. We learned that Sam had had a history of intense fear and avoidance of dogs for three years before this almost tragic interaction. There did not seem to be any obvious triggers for his fear, such as episodes of Sam having been scared or bitten by a dog. Sam was also a shy child. He often hid behind his mother and did not interact well with other children. He became very nervous when anyone would fight at home or school. He often bit his fingernails, complained of stomachaches, and had trouble sleeping most nights. He went through a period during which he complained of being terrorized by monsters in his room. We discovered that one of Sam's grandmothers was a very anxious

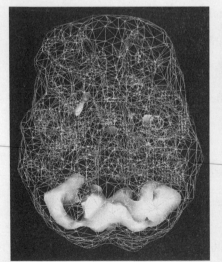 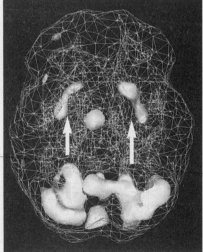

Healthy scan
Good activity in the cerebellum;
cool everywhere else.

Sam's scan
Increased basal ganglia activity.

woman who had panic attacks. She had been addicted to the tranquilizer Valium in the past. Sam also had an uncle who had been excessively shy and had committed suicide at the age of twenty.

Sam's rest and concentration SPECT studies showed markedly increased activity in his basal ganglia. To overcome his fear we used a combination of biofeedback and systematic desensitization and helped him with his negative thoughts.

TESSA

From several vantage points in our office, we are able to see patients in the waiting room before they see us. Sometimes our most important information comes from a few seconds of this type of observation. Tessa, seventeen, looked very uncomfortable and ill at ease. As we watched this pretty, petite teenager, her hands were tremulous, a leg bounced nervously, and her eyes darted around the room. Her parents brought her to our clinic because she was living her life in self-imposed solitary confinement. Unlike other teenage girls, who begin to bond strongly to a peer group, Tessa kept to herself. She avoided talking in class for fear others would think she was stupid. So great

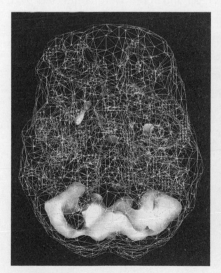 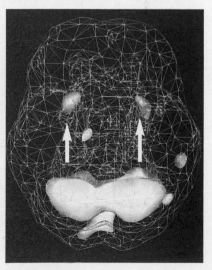

Healthy scan
Good activity in the cerebellum; cool everywhere else.

Tessa's scan
Increased basal ganglia activity.

were her fears of having an accident that learning to drive was simply out of the question. Tessa avoided shopping malls because of an intensely uncomfortable sense that "something bad would happen." She avoided looking for a job for fear of rejection. Teachers thought she was reclusive and other teens thought she was stuck-up. Her grades and school attendance were good. No one knew of her private hell. Tessa had an uncle and a cousin who had been diagnosed with anxiety disorders. Tessa had seen a psychotherapist for several months but did not find it helpful. We ordered a SPECT series on Tessa, which showed markedly increased activity in her basal ganglia at rest and with concentration. Because psychotherapy by itself had not been helpful to Tessa, we decided to put her on an antidepressant to calm her basal ganglia and then teach her biofeedback and other forms of self-relaxation, which over time allowed her to make friends, be more vocal in class, and learn to drive. She was also able to gradually discontinue her medication.

Jesse

Jesse, thirty-nine, a homemaker and mother of three, was assailed with self-doubt and tormented by constant worrying. She second-guessed her every decision. How she disciplined her children, what she wore to the grocery store, the meal she planned for dinner—all and more were connected to a never-ending cycle of anxious thoughts. Jesse found herself obsessing over the details of what her children would think, what the neighbors would think, what her husband would think, and so on. No wonder her upper back was filled with knots of tension and her head frequently felt like it was in a vise. She had trouble relaxing during sex. Not only did Jesse suffer from anxiety, but everyone in the house suffered as well. Initially, her husband tried to be supportive and reassure her, but after several years he withdrew, which led to even more anxiety for Jesse. Ultimately, she and her husband sought the help of a marital therapist, who sent Jesse to see us. Jesse's father had had periods of panic attacks in his life and her mother tended to be a very negative person. Through relaxation training and cognitive therapy, Jesse became more relaxed, more positive, and more connected to her husband and children.

Type 1, Pure Anxiety may respond positively to psychological interventions, such as biofeedback and Automatic Negative Thought (ANT) therapy (or therapy for one's own thoughts), and this may be the only treatment needed.

Nutritional supplements are also frequently used, especially in mild cases. Medications are usually necessary when anxiety is debilitating, as in the case of moderate to severe disorders. They may also be used on a short-term basis to reduce the symptoms so that a patient is comfortable enough to participate in psychological treatments, or they may be the long-term treatment approach. Antidepressants, especially the tricyclic antidepressants desipramine and imipramine, and anticonvulsants are often effective in treating Pure Anxiety. Anti-anxiety medications are occasionally used on a short-term basis in combination with the antidepressants.

Type 2: Pure Depression

Pure Depression results from excessive activity in the brain's emotional center, the deep limbic system. This type is associated with primary depressive symptoms that range from chronic mild sadness (Dysthymia) to the devastating illness of major depression. The hallmark symptoms of Pure Depression include: a persistent sad or negative mood; a loss of interest in usually pleasurable activities; periods of crying; frequent feelings of guilt, helplessness, hopelessness, or worthlessness; sleep and appetite changes (too much or too little); low energy levels; suicidal thoughts or attempts; and low self-esteem. Major Depressive Episode and Dysthymia are examples of illnesses in this category.

The SPECT findings that correlate with Pure Depression are markedly increased activity in the deep limbic area at rest and during concentration, and decreased prefrontal cortex activity at rest that improves with concentration. Deactivation of the prefrontal cortex at rest and improvement with concentration is a finding that is very common but is not always present. The twelve most common symptoms of Type 2, Pure Depression are:

1. Persistent sad or "empty" mood

2. Loss of interest or pleasure in activities that are usually fun, including sex

3. Restlessness, irritability, or excessive crying

4. Feelings of guilt, worthlessness, helplessness, hopelessness, pessimism

5. Sleeping too much or too little, early-morning awakening

6. Appetite and/or weight loss, or overeating and weight gain

7. Decreased energy, fatigue, feeling "slowed down"

8. Thoughts of death or suicide, or suicide attempts

9. Difficulty concentrating, remembering, or making decisions

10. Persistent physical symptoms that do not respond to treatment, such as headaches, digestive disorders, and chronic pain

11. Persistent negativity or chronic low self-esteem

12. Persistent feeling of dissatisfaction or boredom

VICKIE

Vickie was nine years old and she cried every day. Vickie's parents were deeply concerned about her because she never seemed to have fun or experience joy. Vickie's classmates enjoyed things like seeing each other at school, going to the beach, visiting at each other's homes, and taking dance classes, but Vickie had no interest in those things. Dr. Routh found a very sad little girl who sat looking at the floor in the waiting room. Playfully, Dr. Routh tried to establish eye contact with her, and, when she finally did, Vickie's eyes were filled with such sadness that Dr. Routh felt like crying, too. Dr. Routh discovered that Vickie felt school failure was imminent even though she got mostly As and Bs in her classes. Vickie described a sense of being lost and alone when in fact her friends still called looking for her. Most ominously, Vickie believed she was a burden to her family and gave the example of her mother now having to take her to doctors. Every night she had trouble sleeping and often had little appetite. She also had had thoughts of death and suicide for several years, but had just recently begun to share them with her mother. Vickie's mother had suffered from depression after the birth of Vickie's sister, and Vickie's maternal grandmother had periods of depression that put her to bed for weeks at a time. As part of Vickie's evaluation, we performed a brain SPECT series, which revealed marked hyperactivity in her brain's deep limbic system. Additionally, her prefrontal cortex was less active at rest but was better with concentration (a common finding with depression). With a combination of antidepressant medication, education about the nature of her illness using the images of her brain for illustration and cognitive therapy, a sense of happiness and peace returned to Vickie's life and she was able to enjoy herself again.

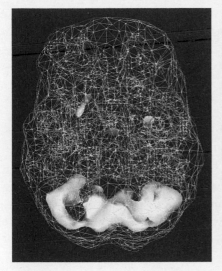 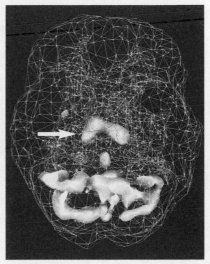

Healthy scan
Good activity in the cerebellum; cool everywhere else.

Vicki's scan
Increased deep limbic (thalamus) activity (arrow).

GEOFFREY

Geoffrey was a happy teenager who excelled in many pursuits—academics, baseball, video games, and attracting girls. Six months after he turned fourteen his mother brought him to our clinic. When we saw him, Geoffrey was not the same guy he had been a few months earlier. He had dropped out of sports, had no interest in his friends, and was having problems at school. He spent most of his time alone in his room with his video games. He cried for little or no reason, developed trouble sleeping at night, and had little appetite. He yelled insults at his parents when they tried to get him involved with friends or family activities, and he most often saw the negative side of his life. His parents brought him to see us after his report card showed he was failing the ninth grade. Geoffrey's father suffered from periods of depression, and he had been addicted to painkilling medication in his twenties. It was clear that Geoffrey suffered from a Major Depressive Episode, what we call Pure Depression. Because, in our opinion, Geoffrey's diagnosis was clear and the family was able to understand the likely underlying problems, we did not order a SPECT series. Depression often presents itself shortly after puberty, due to a change in hormones. With a combination of medication, exercise, dietary changes, and therapy, Geoffrey became his old self once again, did well in school, and became much more social with his friends.

MARY ANN

When Mary Ann, forty-six, came to the clinic, she had felt sad nearly every day for the previous eight months. Almost anything seemed to cause a crying episode; she saw the negative side of most events, and was very irritable toward her boyfriend and daughter. As joy ebbed from her life she lost interest in sex, wondered if she had enough energy to get through her workday, complained of memory problems, and didn't return phone calls from her friends. Because she felt exhausted at the end of the day, Mary Ann related that she could go to sleep easily at night, but almost always woke up about 2:30 A.M. and couldn't get back to sleep. She lost weight, even though she wasn't dieting, and started to think her boyfriend and daughter would be better off if she were dead. At her boyfriend's insistence, she came to see us. Her SPECT series showed markedly increased activity in her deep limbic system on both her resting and concentration studies. At rest, there was less activity in her prefrontal cortex. Seeing her scan helped Mary Ann realize that her bad feelings were not her fault. She wanted to try a natural supplement before medication, because she worried about side effects. We put her on SAMe, an exercise regimen, and therapy. Within three weeks she started to feel much better. She was more positive with her daughter, more affectionate with her boyfriend, happier, and more energetic. A follow-up scan six months later showed significant calming of her emotional brain.

Type 2, Pure Depression should be treated with antidepressant medications if it is severe. Mild cases may be treated with supplements. It is also very important to incorporate the use of other interventions, such as therapy, diet and exercise, education, and support groups. Medications or supplements are rarely the sole answer to the problem. Treatment of Pure Depression is not a short-term or hit-or-miss event and should not be undertaken lightly. This applies not only to medication management, but also to the use of herbs and supplements, diet and exercise strategies, and psychotherapy interventions. A single episode of Pure Depression should be treated continuously for a year. Two episodes of Pure Depression should be treated continuously for three years. Three or more episodes should be treated for life. We address treatment for Pure Depression in more detail in chapter 7.

Type 3: Mixed Anxiety and Depression

Sufferers of this type have a combination of both Pure Anxiety symptoms and Pure Depression symptoms. This type shows excessive activity in the brain's basal ganglia and the deep limbic system. One type may predominate at any point in time, but both symptom clusters are present on a regular basis.

KEENAN

Keenan, five, appeared sad and tense when his mother and father brought him to see us. Keenan's constant whining drove his parents to distraction. He never seemed happy like their other two children. He experienced no joy in learning something new, and most things were a struggle. It was a battle to get Keenan out of bed in the morning; a battle to get him to eat breakfast; a battle to get him dressed; and a battle to get him off to school. At night, the family braced itself for another siege and battled to get Keenan to eat dinner, pick up his room, brush his teeth, and go to bed. Keenan constantly bit his fingernails and toenails to the point where they bled. He complained of frequent headaches and tummy aches. And he always seemed to predict the worst, saying no one at school liked him, he would never learn to catch a ball, and he wouldn't be able to learn to read like his brother and sister. Negativity and anxiety were an everyday part of Keenan's young life. His grandmother had been hospitalized for depression and on one occasion had been treated with electroshock therapy. Keenan had seen a psychologist but this had not seemed to help. His pediatrician also had tried him on an antidepressant and again, his parents didn't notice much improvement. We ordered a SPECT series to better understand Keenan. The SPECT series showed markedly increased activity in his deep limbic system and left basal ganglia on both studies that was worse when Keenan concentrated. Treatment consisted of antidepressant medication to calm Keenan's basal ganglia and deep limbic system, exercise, and parent training to help his parents more effectively deal with his difficult behavior.

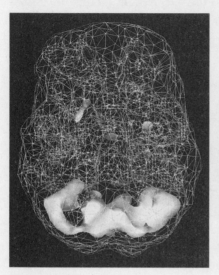 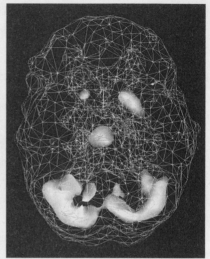

Healthy scan
Good activity in the cerebellum;
cool everywhere else.

Keenan's scan
Increased activity in the left basal
ganglia and the deep limbic system.

JULIANNE

Julianne, sixteen, was brought to our clinic because she was failing in school. She had done well until the seventh grade, but then started having problems with erratic performance. Her parents said that she appeared depressed. Her teachers said she was withdrawn and rarely participated in class. Julianne complained that she never felt right. "I feel nervous and sad most of the time. I am never comfortable in my own skin," she said. "I never talk in class, my heart races when I think of raising my hand. If I have an assignment where I have to give an oral presentation, I stay home sick from school. I just can't do it." Julianne had smoked marijuana on a number of occasions, which she said helped her feel calm inside. Julianne bit and picked her fingernails to such an extent that her mother started taking her for manicures to see if that would help her break the habit. Her SPECT series showed in-

Julianne's SPECT Scans

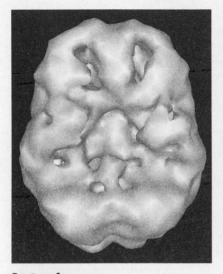

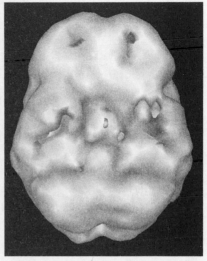

Rest surface scan
Scalloping (bumpiness—drug exposure) and decreased prefrontal cortex activity at rest.

Concentration surface scan
Scalloping and improved prefrontal activity with concentration.

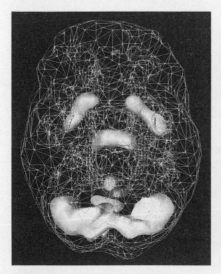

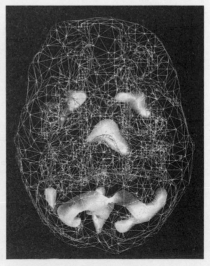

Rest active scan
Increased basal ganglia and deep limbic activity.

Concentration active scan
Increased basal ganglia and deep limbic activity.

creased basal ganglia and deep limbic activity on both studies and decreased prefrontal cortex activity at rest that improved with concentration. In addition, there was mild scalloping across the cortical surface of the scan, likely indicating toxic exposure from the marijuana use. We helped Julianne understand that she was using marijuana as a form of medication to calm her anxiety, but she had no idea it was hurting her brain. The scan helped her to stop using marijuana and cooperate with treatment, which included a combination of medication, biofeedback, and cognitive therapy.

MIKE

Mike, fifty-eight, was filled with anxiety throughout most days. As a project manager at a software company in the Silicon Valley, he was concerned that he wouldn't be able to keep up with the younger people at work. He tended to predict failure for himself and the projects on which he worked. He had many headaches, felt tense in his neck and shoulders, and had been to the emergency room several times that year for chest pain that was eventually diagnosed as anxiety. Mike also felt moody and negative. He had trouble sleeping most nights, and experienced little pleasure in life. His wife had divorced him because she said he was too negative and they never had any fun together. Mike drank heavily at night to calm his nerves. When his boss became concerned about Mike's work performance, he referred him to the clinic. Mike's SPECT series showed markedly increased basal ganglia and deep limbic activity on both studies and decreased prefrontal cortex activity at rest that improved with concentration. Mike's scans also showed significant scalloping across the cortical surface of his brain. This finding was likely related to the toxic levels of alcohol Mike was using. We explained to Mike that he was using alcohol as a form of medication to calm his anxiety, but, like Julianne, he had no idea it was hurting his brain. The scan helped him stop using alcohol and engage with treatment, which included a combination of medication, alcohol counseling, biofeedback, and cognitive therapy.

Type 3, Mixed Anxiety and Depression is best treated with psychological interventions targeted at both anxiety and depression, such as biofeedback, interpersonal psychotherapy, and cognitive therapy, as well as antidepressant medications or supplements that have a calming effect on the basal ganglia and the deep limbic areas. Any potentially toxic substances used in self-medication, such as mood-altering drugs or alcohol, must be stopped for treatment to be effective.

Type 4: Overfocused Anxiety/Depression

Overfocused Anxiety/Depression results from excessive activity in the brain's anterior cingulate gyrus, the basal ganglia, and/or the deep limbic system. The anterior cingulate gyrus is the brain's gear shifter. When there is too much activity in the anterior cingulate gyrus, people cannot shift their attention properly and end up stuck on negative thoughts or behaviors. When this is combined with excessive basal ganglia activity, people get stuck on anxious thoughts. When this is combined with excessive deep limbic activity, people get stuck on negative, depressing thoughts. Many people get stuck on both anxiety-provoking and depressive thoughts. Obsessive-Compulsive Disorder (stuck on negative thoughts or actions), phobias (stuck on a fear), eating disorders (stuck on negative eating behavior), and Posttraumatic Stress Disorder (PTSD, stuck on a past traumatic event) fit into this type. This type is also associated with people who worry, tend to hold grudges, and have problems with oppositional or argumentative behavior. We have also noticed that this type tends to occur more frequently in children or grandchildren of alcoholics. SPECT findings that are associated with this type show increased anterior cingulate gyrus activity and increased basal ganglia and/or deep limbic activity at rest and during concentration. Sometimes there is markedly increased activity in the anterior cingulate gyrus with concentration; other times it calms a bit with concentration.

When anterior cingulate gyrus hyperactivity becomes worse with concentration, it usually means that, as this person tries to focus on something, he or she becomes more anxious or more stuck in negative thoughts or behaviors. The more intensely they concentrate, the worse the problem becomes. Finding ways to take a break from these negative situations or to disrupt the repetitive thought patterns can be very helpful.

Symptoms of Type 4, Overfocused Anxiety/Depression include at least four items from the Pure Anxiety (page 47) and/or Pure Depression (page 51) checklists, plus at least four of the following:

1. Excessive or senseless worrying

2. Upset when things are out of place or don't go the way you planned

3. Tendency to be oppositional or argumentative

4. Tendency to have repetitive negative or anxious thoughts

5. Tendency toward compulsive or addictive behaviors

6. Intense dislike of change

7. Tendency to hold grudges

8. Difficulty seeing options in situations

9. Tendency to hold on to own opinion and not listen to others

10. Need to have things done a certain way or you become very upset

11. Others complain that you worry too much

12. Tend to say no without first thinking about question

KATIE

Katie was brought to our clinic for tantrums that were out of control. She was defiant, argumentative, and very negative. She took no delight in activities that other seven-year-old children enjoy and was extremely fearful of being left with anyone besides her mother. She worried about the doors being locked at night and she had to wash her hands several times before each meal to keep the germs away. She was afraid to sleep in her bed and was adept at forcing her way into her parents' bed. When things did not go the way she expected she would cry and carry on for hours. Teachers complained about her behavior and she had few friends because she was so bossy. On her seventh birthday, her parents surprised her by taking her to Disneyland. Because she didn't know about it ahead of time, she threw a tantrum in the Disneyland parking lot. It was two hours before her parents could calm her down and go into the park. Katie's parents initially gave in to her demands in an attempt to soothe her and stop the tantrums. They soon realized that this didn't work. By giving in, Katie's parents were actually making her behavior worse. Katie appeared to be resistant to any form of discipline. Spanking didn't help, lectures seemed worthless, and no amount of praise was helpful. Her mother had grown up in an alcoholic home and struggled with issues of anxiety and depression. Katie also had an uncle who had Obsessive-Compulsive Disorder.

Katie's SPECT series showed markedly increased anterior cingulate gyrus, basal ganglia, and deep limbic activity on her concentration and baseline scans. Activity in the anterior cingulate gyrus increased during concentration. The scans helped Katie's parents gain a better understanding of her problems and follow-through with treatment. Katie's treatment included St. John's wort, a natural herbal supplement, biofeedback for self-control, and an exercise regimen. Additionally, through parent training we helped her parents be more effective with her. The treatment helped Katie relax and feel happier and less anxious, and over time she became more compliant. A follow-up concentration scan several months later showed nice improvement.

Katie's Before and After Treatment

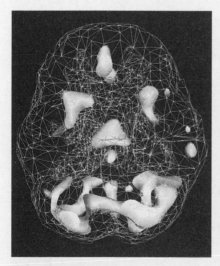 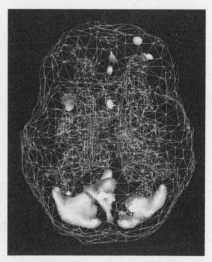

Before treatment
Increased anterior cingulate gyrus, BG, and DLS activity.

After treatment
Overall calming of the anterior cingulate gyrus, BG, and DLS.

MARK

Mark, fifteen, was one of those teenagers who make even professionals nervous. He appeared full of hatred and rage. In the waiting room he gave Dr. Amen a look that said, "Doc, you are just wasting your time and my parents' money. You can't help me." He had trouble with most authority figures and was frequently kicked out of class for talking back to teachers. Mark also had problems with depression, worry, and anxiety. He was stubborn and willful. There was daily turmoil between Mark and his parents. We were the fourth clinic at which his parents had sought help. A number of therapists had said that there was nothing they could do for Mark until he changed his attitude. Individual psychotherapy, family therapy, and tough-love parent training had been ineffective. A number of medications also were ineffective. The year before we saw him, Mark had started using alcohol and marijuana. He said it made him feel happier and more relaxed inside. Mark's father had been diagnosed with alcohol abuse in his early twenties. Mark's paternal grandfather and several uncles also had had trouble with drugs, alcohol, or both.

Mark's SPECT series showed markedly increased anterior cingulate gyrus, basal ganglia, and deep limbic activity, which was worse during concentration. The scans helped his parents understand Mark's negative attitude and helped us direct treatment for him. Mark was placed on a serotonergic antidepressant to calm the anterior cingulate gyrus part of his brain. He and his parents also saw a family counselor to help them communicate more effectively. The treatment helped Mark be more cooperative and feel happier and less anxious.

LEIGH ANN

Leigh Ann, thirty-two, was obsessed with her ex-boyfriend. She could not get him out of her head, although they had only dated for several months. She cried day and night, called him repeatedly, and felt intense anxiety longing for him. She couldn't sleep at night, suffered tension headaches and neck pain, and couldn't relax. A part of her knew the obsession was stupid, but she couldn't control herself. Leigh Ann's job performance at a nearby brewery became very erratic. She yelled at coworkers and started to call in sick. Her employee assistance worker called us for help. Leigh Ann's SPECT series showed markedly increased activity in the anterior cingulate gyrus, basal ganglia, and deep limbic system, and these findings worsened with concentration.

Initially, Leigh Ann did not talk to us about her obsession with her ex-boyfriend. She complained of chronic anxiety, depression, and worrying. As she felt better with the treatment, which consisted of a serotonergic antidepressant, relaxation training, and cognitive therapy, she was able to form a more trusting relationship with her therapist and was able to begin dealing with underlying issues. The treatment helped her calm the repetitive thoughts and move beyond the relationship.

Type 4, Overfocused Anxiety/Depression is best treated with interventions that increase the neurotransmitter serotonin. Treatment can include medication, such as selective serotonin reuptake inhibitors (SSRIs) and antidepressants (Prozac, Zoloft, Celexa, or Paxil); dietary changes; natural supplements, such as 5-HTP and St. John's wort; and intense aerobic exercise. We do not use natural supplements with antidepressants as it may overload the system with serotonin. Behavior therapy has also been shown to calm these parts of the brain. For severe cases we use the atypical antipsychotic medications, such as Risperdal and Zyprexa, and in the most resistant cases some physicians have performed neurosurgery to cut the connections to and from the anterior cingulate gyrus (called a cingulatomy).

Type 5: Cyclic Anxiety/Depression

Cyclic Anxiety/Depression results from excessive focal activity in the brain's basal ganglia and/or deep limbic system. These focal "hot" areas in the brain act like "emotional seizures" as the emotional centers hijack the brain for periods of time. Like typical seizures, patients have little or no control over these episodes. Cyclic disorders, such as Bipolar Disorder, Cyclothymia, and Premenstrual Dysphoric Disorder (PMDD), along with panic attacks, fit in this category because they are episodic and unpredictable. The hallmark of Type 5 is its cyclic nature. Not surprisingly, SPECT scan findings vary with the phase of the illness or point in the patient's cycle. For example, when someone is in a manic phase of a bipolar illness there is increased focal deep limbic activity and patchy increased uptake (multiple focal hot spots) throughout the brain; when this same person is in a depressed state there is increased focal deep limbic activity but it is often associated with overall decreased activity (no patchy increased uptake). Similarly, a woman with Premenstrual Dysphoric Disorder may show only increased focal deep limbic activity during the unaffected time of her cycle, but show increased focal deep limbic activity, decreased prefrontal cortex, and increased anterior cingulate gyrus activity during the worst time of her cycle.

Like the other types, Cyclic Anxiety/Depression is a spectrum disorder, which means that one can have a very mild or a very severe form, or anything in between. One may have mild PMS, or a mild cyclic mood disorder, or the problems can be so severe as to be life threatening. Cyclic Anxiety/Depression must be closely and skillfully monitored, especially at critical times in the course of the disorder—for instance, when medications are first started—because antidepressants may trigger mania; at hormonal transition times, when a patient is experiencing additional intense stressors; and in the case of a medically fragile individual. If the problem interferes with your life, you need professional treatment.

The hallmark of this type is a cyclic pattern of anxiety or depression. Symptoms of this type include at least four items from the Pure Anxiety (page 47) and/or Pure Depression (page 51) checklists, plus at least four of the following:

1. Periods of abnormally elevated, depressed, or anxious mood

2. Periods of decreased need for sleep, feeling energetic on dramatically less sleep than usual

3. Periods of grandiose notions, ideas, or plans

4. Periods of increased talking or pressured speech

5. Periods of too many thoughts racing through the mind

6. Periods of markedly increased energy

7. Periods of poor judgment that lead to risk-taking behavior (separate from usual behavior)

8. Periods of inappropriate social behavior

9. Periods of irritability or aggression

10. Periods of delusional or psychotic thinking

ERIC

Eric, eight, had terrible mood swings. He had periods when he was sweet and gentle that alternated with times of intense irritability and anger. It was hard to predict what mood he would be in on any given day. His school performance also alternated; some days he was focused and easily finished all of his work; other days he dawdled for hours, couldn't concentrate, and was off task. Eric had been diagnosed with Attention Deficit Hyperactivity Disorder (ADHD) by his pediatrician and placed on Ritalin. Unfortunately, it made him dramatically more irritable and his parents stopped the medication after two weeks. His parents brought him to us after a particularly irritable mood that lasted several weeks. During this episode he had lost friends at school and alienated his baseball teammates with his temper outbursts. Eric's paternal grandmother had been diagnosed with manic depressive illness (now called Bipolar Disorder) and had spent time in a state psychiatric hospital. Eric's father suffered from periods of depression.

Eric's SPECT study showed a focal "hot area" in his deep limbic system and also marked increased activity throughout the cortex of the brain. The pattern is one we call the "ring of fire," because it looks like a ring of hyperactivity around the brain. He was diagnosed with a cyclic mood disorder (likely early Bipolar Disorder) and placed on an antiseizure medication to calm the overactive area. Over the next few weeks his mood stabilized and he became more even-tempered.

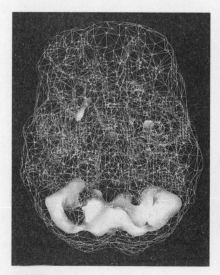 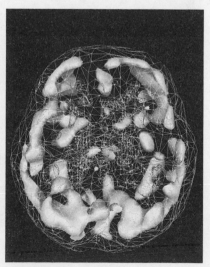

Healthy scan
Good activity in the cerebellum;
cool everywhere else.

Eric's scan
Increased left basal ganglia
and deep limbic system activity.

KENDALL

Kendall's moodiness started at puberty. Before the age of thirteen, when her menstrual cycle started, she was an even-tempered child. After thirteen, she started to go through major mood swings. The two weeks before her period were filled with sad feelings, negativity, and irritability. At these times she craved sugar, struggled with sleep, and felt surges of anxiety. Everyone in her family tracked her menstrual cycle because they all were affected by the "other Kendall," as she was labeled during these times. Her symptoms subsided two to three days after she started her period. She was seventeen when she came to our clinic. In the previous year she had gone through six boyfriends—she tended to break up with them during the premenstrual periods.

Kendall had two SPECT studies as part of her evaluation: one several days before the onset of her menstrual period (during the worst time of her cycle) and one a week after her menstrual period started (during the best time of her cycle). They were dramatically different. During the worst time of her cycle there was a large focal hot spot in her deep limbic area. During

Kendall's Scans

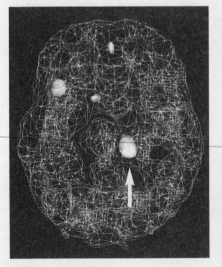 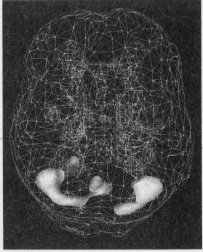

Before-period scan
Increased focal deep limbic activity (arrow).

After-period scan
Overall improvement.

the best time in her cycle the spot was much less intense. She was diagnosed with a cyclic mood disorder (severe Premenstrual Dysphoric Disorder) and placed on an antiseizure medication to calm the overactive area. Her emotional state during her cycles improved dramatically over the next few months.

SARAH

Sarah was fifty-three years old when she was admitted to the hospital under Dr. Amen's care. One month prior, her family had had her committed to another psychiatric hospital for delusional thinking and bizarre behavior— she had ripped out all the electrical wiring in her home because she heard voices coming from the walls. She was barely getting any sleep, her thoughts raced wildly, and she was irritable. In the previous hospital, her doctor had diagnosed her with Bipolar Disorder (a cyclical mood disorder). He had placed her on lithium (an anti-manic medication) and an anti-anxiety medication. After responding well, she was sent home. Sarah did not want to believe that anything was wrong with her and she stopped taking both medications. Some members of her family endorsed her actions and told her she didn't need pills because doctors only prescribe them to force patients into numerous follow-up visits. Their advice was ill advised, for within weeks of stopping the treatment Sarah's bizarre behavior returned. When Dr. Amen first saw Sarah, she was extremely paranoid. Believing that everyone was trying to hurt her, she was always looking for ways to escape the hospital. Her thoughts became delusional; she believed she had special powers that others were trying to take away from her. At times she also appeared very "spacey." A SPECT study was ordered.

Carrying this out was not easy. The clinic tried to scan her on three separate occasions. The first two times she ripped out the intravenous line, accusing us of trying to poison her. The third time was a success because her sister was with her and calmed her down by talking her through the experience. The study revealed increased focal deep limbic uptake and a marked patchy uptake across the cortex. For Sarah's family, this was powerful evidence that her problems were biological, so that when she refused medication they were now willing to encourage her to go back on it. On medication her behavior normalized again and she felt better and more in control. When she was better she was shown her scan and the biological basis for her need for medication. Through a better understanding of the problem, she agreed to follow-up visits and to stay on her medication.

Sarah's case illustrates one of the most clinically significant problems encountered with people diagnosed with bipolar illness. This disorder is usually quite responsive to medication. The problem is that when people afflicted by the disorder improve, they feel so normal they do not believe they ever had a problem to begin with and are even more reluctant to accept that they have a chronic illness. It is difficult for people to accept that they have to keep taking medication when they think they no longer have a problem. Yet, as we have seen, prematurely stopping medication actually increases the chances for relapse. Through the use of these brain studies we have been able to decrease the relapse rate of our patients by demonstrating graphically the biological nature of their disorders and the need to treat them as such. It has been a great asset to us in getting patients to cooperate in their own healing process. In addition, it has helped us convince patients to stop blaming themselves for their symptoms.

Type 5, Cyclic Anxiety/Depression is best treated with mood stabilizers such as lithium or anticonvulsant medications. Dietary omega-3 fatty acids can also be helpful, as can the amino acid gamma-laminobutyric acid (GABA). Psychological interventions can also help decrease the stressors that may trigger an episode of the disorder. Antidepressant therapy may be necessary, but, as we said previously, this needs to be very closely monitored because of the risk of triggering mania.

Seasonal Affective Disorder: A Variant of Type 5

The turkey is roasting in the oven, the fall days have grown crisp with the first hint of winter, and everyone is excitedly waiting for Thanksgiving guests to arrive for dinner—everyone except those suffering from Seasonal Affective Disorder (SAD). People with SAD are not energized by the Indian summer days of fall and do not look forward to the holiday season with joyful anticipation. Instead, they begin to experience the annual onset of the symptoms of this variant of cyclic depression.

SAD is similar in many ways to recurrent Major Depressive Disorder; however it may have more atypical features. Atypical features are oversleeping as opposed to insomnia, weight gain and increased appetite rather than weight loss and loss of appetite, and agitation instead of feeling slowed down. People with SAD feel run-down, irritable, and depressed. They have increased appetite, especially for carbohydrates, and usually gain weight. They also feel like they never get enough rest even though they are sleeping more than usual. Some describe themselves as feeling like a grouchy bear that needs to hibernate during the winter.

The holiday season is difficult for many people. Financial pressures and the expectations of family members are great. For those of us who have lost a loved one or are alone, grief reactions can be intense during the holidays. Typically, the "holiday blues" resolve rapidly with social support or without intervention after the first of the year. SAD, on the other hand, continues to intensify during the holiday season, the winter months, and into early spring. Without intervention, the symptoms do not begin to abate until early to mid spring, or until summertime for some patients, when the days are longer.

The most likely explanation for the cause of SAD is light deprivation. Sunlight detected by the retina of the eye sends signals to the more primitive parts of the brain, one of which is the pineal gland. The pineal gland plays a vital role in hormone regulation, and one of the hormones it controls is melatonin. Melatonin, in turn, helps set the body's biorhythms. Disruption of the pineal gland hormonal axis is thought to be a primary cause of SAD. Support for this line of thought comes from several observations. First, SAD is decidedly more common in parts of the world that are more deprived of sunlight. In the United States, the rate of SAD is much higher in the Pacific Northwest and in Maine than in Ohio, and the rate is highest in Alaska. The rate of SAD is higher in Scandinavian countries than in southern European countries. Second, people with SAD who travel to a more southern location experience improvement in their symptoms. Third, the development of bright light therapy, discussed below, has proved beneficial for SAD patients who are not fully responsive to other forms of treatment.

Children are not immune to SAD. In fact some of us who have a great deal of experience with SAD (Dr. Routh practiced in Alaska for several years and continues to consult there) believe children may be more vulnerable to the disorder. Native Alaskans have a high rate of SAD, which may come as a surprise to many people who may assume that Native Alaskans should be used to light deprivation since they have lived for generations in such an environment. Once again, those of us who have lived with and worked with this population have observed that these populations have undergone tremendous changes in their social structures in the past two generations, and consequently protective mechanisms against mental illnesses including SAD have broken down.

We have written about the many variations of depression and anxiety disorders and there are variant forms of SAD as well. Some individuals living in the very hot regions of the United States experience the onset of depressive symptoms in the summertime and feel better in the winter. For these people, the trigger is not light deprivation but too much heat or possibly light.

Many people with SAD respond to antidepressants. Because they tend to have atypical symptoms of overeating and weight gain, fatigue, feeling rundown, and an increased need for sleep, they usually respond best to an antidepressant that either helps with appetite control or at least doesn't increase their appetite. Therefore, those of us who treat SAD patients prescribe Wellbutrin or an SSRI like Prozac. These two antidepressants can be used alone or in combination and combined with medications for the treatment of anxiety disorders or with anticonvulsants/mood stabilizers. There are some patients with SAD who don't fully respond to treatment regardless of which antidepressant is used. They get better, but they don't get well. These patients are the ones who typically need sunlight. Unfortunately, most insurance companies won't pay for therapeutic trips to Hawaii even though in many cases a trip would cost less than ongoing treatment. Most people are not in a position to move to the Southwest or Texas or Florida on "doctor's orders," either, so we prescribe bright light therapy.

Tanning beds do not provide bright light therapy. If you try to treat your SAD by going for tanning booth sessions, it won't work. You'll ruin your skin, get wrinkles earlier, and only give yourself more reasons to be depressed. Bright light therapy is full-spectrum light and it has to be at least 10,000 lux or higher to be effective. "Full spectrum" is important terminology; it means that the light is the same color spectrum as sunlight. Other types of light won't do for the treatment of SAD. How the light is used is also extremely important. Overhead lights won't work nor will any of those gimmicks you see in magazines like lights in visors or hats. Full-spectrum light panel boxes (10,000 lux or higher) need to be placed close enough for you to get intense exposure, and this means two to four feet from your eyes and at eye level. You need to be in the presence of the light for an hour every morning, and you may need another hour in the afternoon as well. Periodically during the hour that you sit with the light, you need to glance at it for a few seconds so that it stimulates the retina and sends signals to your brain. You can read, cook, or watch TV as long as you remember to look at the light.

Many people have a dramatic response to bright light therapy. Light therapy can be used alone or in combination with medication to boost its effectiveness.

Type 6: Temporal Lobe Anxiety/Depression

Temporal Lobe Anxiety/Depression results from too much or too little activity in the brain's temporal lobes, in addition to too much activity in the basal ganglia and/or deep limbic system. The temporal lobes are very important to memory, moods, and emotions. When there are problems in this part of the brain, people struggle with temper outbursts, memory problems, mood instability, visual or auditory illusions, and dark, frightening, or evil thoughts. People with this type tend to misinterpret comments as negative when they are not, have trouble reading social situations, and appear to have mild paranoia. They may also have episodes of panic or fear for no specific reason, experience frequent periods of déjà vu, and be preoccupied with religious thoughts. People with this type are the most likely to exhibit aggressive behaviors toward others or themselves. There may be a family history of these problems or they can be triggered by a brain injury. SPECT findings in Type 6 patients show increased or decreased activity in the temporal lobes and increased basal ganglia and/or deep limbic activity at rest and during concentration. When the temporal lobes become less active with concentration, people often struggle with learning problems. When they are less active on the left side there is a tendency toward reading problems and irritability; when they are less active on the right side there is a tendency to have trouble reading social situations. It is possible to have decreased activity on both sides.

This type of anxiety/depression may be aggravated by serotonergic antidepressants. When Dr. Amen first started imaging work in the early 1990s, there was significant media coverage about the controversy that certain antidepressants classified as SSRIs actually made some people more aggressive. The headlines indicated that medications like Prozac, the mother of SSRI medication, made some people more aggressive and more suicidal. However, a large amount of literature exists supporting the use of SSRI medications, and Prozac in particular, as a primary treatment for aggression. Our overall experience is that when these medications are prescribed properly they can have a dramatically positive effect and they have saved many lives. But we have both had patients who became dramatically worse on these medications. The scan data help us understand which patients may be at risk for this problem. Our experience is that patients with temporal lobe abnormalities and certain patients who have cyclic mood disorders are the ones at greater risk. When a temporal lobe abnormality exists, patients are often at greater risk for a negative reaction to SSRI medication.

Symptoms of this type include at least four items from the Pure Anxiety (page 47) and/or Pure Depression (page 51) checklists, plus at least four of the following:

1. Short fuse or periods of extreme irritability

2. Periods of rage with little provocation

3. Often misinterprets comments as negative when they are not

4. Periods of spaciness or confusion

5. Periods of panic and/or fear for no specific reason

6. Visual or auditory changes, such as seeing shadows or hearing muffled sounds

7. Frequent periods of déjà vu (feeling of being somewhere you have never been)

8. Sensitivity or mild paranoia

9. Headaches or abdominal pain of uncertain origin

10. History of a head injury or family history of violence or explosiveness

11. Dark thoughts that may involve suicidal or homicidal thoughts

12. Periods of forgetfulness or memory problems

STACEY

Stacey, nine, was a very sad girl. Her parents brought her to the clinic because of her frequent talk about death. Stacey struggled in school and also had trouble getting along with other children. She annoyed other kids, got into their space, and generally didn't fit in, leaving her without friends. Stacey's temper outbursts at home were increasing. The outbursts started unpredictably and escalated rapidly, and she was always remorseful afterward.

She had surges of panic that seemed to come from out of the blue. She said she often had the feeling people were following her. Stacey's mother hoped that St. John's wort would alleviate Stacey's anxiety and negativity, but instead it seemed to make her much more irritable. Right before she came to see us she drew pictures of herself hanging from a tree and said she saw images of the devil. Also, there was a family history of severe depression in her mother's father, who had tried to kill himself several times.

Suspecting a left temporal lobe problem, a SPECT series was ordered, which showed markedly decreased left temporal lobe activity on both studies, in addition to increased basal ganglia and deep limbic activity. On her concentration study, Stacey had a focal hot area on the outside of her left temporal lobe complicating the deactivation in this area. Stacey needed an antiseizure medication to stabilize her temporal lobes and to help with mood, anxiety, and irritability. As these target symptoms came under better control, an antidepressant was added to further improve her mood. Another benefit of treatment was that Stacey was able to become better at handling social situations; she started to make friends and did better at school.

BILLY

Billy, fifteen, came to the clinic after he was arrested for exploding a homemade bomb in his neighbor's yard. A year earlier, Billy's parents would never have thought their son capable of such an activity, but he'd changed. Over several months, Billy had grown negative, anxious, and distrustful of others. He had frightening fits of temper. Once, during an argument with his parents, he grabbed a knife and asked them if they wanted him to stab himself. For the first time in his life he started to struggle in school, and he withdrew from his friends.

As part of his evaluation, a SPECT series was ordered. It showed markedly decreased left and right temporal lobe activity on both studies, in addition to increased basal ganglia and deep limbic activity. Billy needed antiseizure medication to help stabilize his mood and decrease his anxiety and irritability. He also needed an antidepressant to help raise his mood. As part of the treatment, he and his parents went to family therapy. Over several months Billy, and his family, began to heal.

ALLISON

Allison, thirty-two, was a senior editor at a book publisher. Although she did brilliant work, others in her department avoided her. She was labeled "the buzz saw" because of her vicious temper. After an embarrassing public display of temper, the publisher insisted she get help. Allison reported that her uncontrollable temper had begun at the age of twenty, after she was involved in a car accident. She was stopped at a light when another car struck her from the left side. The left side of her head broke the driver's-side window. Although she was only briefly unconscious, she said she felt dazed for weeks. Allison also complained of relationship problems, moodiness, and intense periods of anxiety and anger.

Suspecting a brain injury to her left temporal lobe, a SPECT series was ordered. It showed marked decreased left and right temporal lobe activity and increased deep limbic activity on both studies. An antiseizure medication helped to stabilize her mood and calm her anxiety and temper.

Allison's Scan

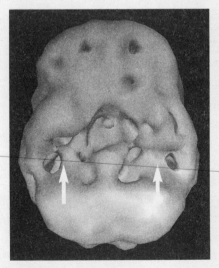 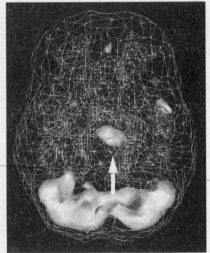

Underside surface view
Decreased left and right temporal lobe activity (arrows).

Underside active view
Increased deep limbic activity (arrow).

Type 6, Temporal Lobe Anxiety/Depression is best treated with a combination of anticonvulsant and antidepressant medications. Psychological interventions, such as interpersonal psychotherapy and cognitive therapy, can be helpful, along with neurofeedback over the temporal lobes.

Type 7: Unfocused Anxiety/Depression

Unfocused Anxiety/Depression results from too little activity in the brain's prefrontal cortex, in addition to excessive activity in the basal ganglia and/or deep limbic system. The prefrontal cortex acts as the brain's supervisor. It helps with executive functions such as attention span, forethought, impulse control, organization, motivation, and planning. When the prefrontal cortex is underactive, people complain of being inattentive, distracted, bored, off task, and impulsive.

This type is often seen in conjunction with another psychiatric illness called Attention Deficit Disorder. ADD, also called ADHD (Attention Deficit Hyperactivity Disorder), is a developmental disorder that starts in childhood and is associated with long-standing issues of short attention span, distractibility, disorganization, restlessness, and impulsivity. Sometimes distinguishing ADD from Unfocused Anxiety/Depression can be difficult, and many feel the distinction is arbitrary. ADD, like depression and anxiety, has a number of subtypes that help to guide treatment. ADD in its classic form starts in childhood and can be seen consistently throughout a person's life. Unfocused Anxiety/Depression may not start until much later in life. Often the two run together. The medication treatments are similar. Unfocused Anxiety/Depression SPECT findings show decreased activity in the prefrontal cortex at rest and during concentration along with increased basal ganglia and/or deep limbic activity.

Symptoms of Unfocused Anxiety/Depression include at least four items from the Pure Anxiety (page 47) and/or Pure Depression (page 51) checklists, plus at least four of the following:

1. Trouble staying focused

2. Spaciness or feeling in a fog

3. Overwhelmed by tasks of daily living

4. Feeling tired, sluggish, or slow-moving

5. Procrastination, failure to finish things

6. Chronic boredom

7. Loses things

8. Easily distracted

9. Forgetful

10. Poor planning skills

11. Difficulty expressing feelings

12. Difficulty expressing empathy for others

CHRIS

Chris, seven, came to see us because he had severe problems with anxiety and depression. He was afraid to leave his mother and often cried for seemingly little or no reason. He frequently appeared distracted and off task at school and had been diagnosed with borderline mental retardation with an IQ of 68. He had trouble paying attention when his father read to him at night. His room was always messy unless his mother organized it for him. Chris's parents did not know that his learning problems were related to his emotional problems and took him to see their family doctor, who prescribed Paxil. Paxil is an SSRI antidepressant medication that is often helpful for anxiety, but it didn't help Chris. His learning problems seemed to worsen.

His parents brought him to our clinic after seeing Dr. Amen interviewed on CNN. As part of his evaluation a brain SPECT series was ordered. It showed significantly decreased activity in his prefrontal cortex and increased basal ganglia and deep limbic activity on both studies. As opposed to an SSRI, which is helpful for Overfocused Anxiety/Depression, Chris was placed on the stimulating antidepressant Wellbutrin. In our experience, Wellbutrin helps to activate the prefrontal cortex and calm the basal ganglia and deep limbic areas. Wellbutrin helped Chris focus better in school and helped calm his anxiety and enhance his mood. In addition, Chris was taught self-calming techniques and how to kill the negative thoughts that invaded his emotional space. A year later his IQ was retested and it jumped from 68 to 105. His ability to learn increased because he could pay attention and use the full function of his prefrontal cortex.

JANIS

Janis's mother brought her to see us because she was worried about Janis's tendency to avoid large gatherings and also to put off anyone who tried to befriend her. She appeared anxious, depressed, and negative. Janis, nineteen, was struggling in junior college. She had never done well in school, even though her IQ was normal. Since childhood Janis had had trouble paying attention, frequently missed assignment deadlines, and was very disorganized. She also had very low self-esteem. "I can never be as smart as the other kids in my classes," she said, and she had a strong tendency to put herself down. She told us that she had a strong internal critic. She said, "The voices inside my head always seem mad at me." Her younger brother had been diagnosed with ADD and was taking stimulant medication.

As part of her evaluation a brain SPECT series was ordered. It showed increased basal ganglia and deep limbic activity on both studies and decreased prefrontal cortex activity on both studies that became worse with concentration. Janis was placed on Wellbutrin, which helped her anxiety and mood and also seemed to help her in school. Adderall, a commonly prescribed stimulant medication, was subsequently added and further improved her concentration. Janis also followed our recommendations to start an exercise program, eat more protein, and learn self-calming and negative-thought-killing techniques.

ROBERT

Robert, forty-six, came to the clinic at the insistence of his wife. She was ready to leave him unless he got help. He was negative, anxious, irritable, and very disorganized. He complained of very low energy levels (even though after testing, his medical doctor said there was nothing wrong), and he had no motivation. He hated his job, but did nothing to change the situation. He failed to finish projects that he started and frequently forgot to do the tasks that his wife had asked him to do.

As part of his evaluation a brain SPECT series was ordered. It showed increased basal ganglia and deep limbic activity on both studies and decreased prefrontal cortex activity on both studies that was worse on the concentration study. Robert was placed on Wellbutrin, which helped his anxiety and mood and also seemed to help him have better energy, focus, and achievement. Work was easier to tolerate and his employer was happier

Janis's SPECT Scans

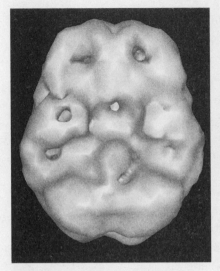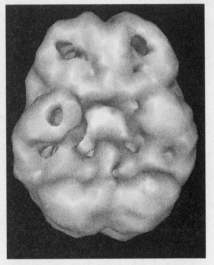

Rest surface scan

Concentration surface scan

Decreased prefrontal cortex activity, seen on both studies, worse with concentration.

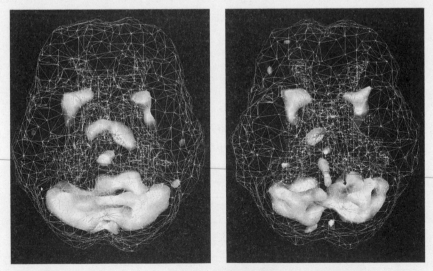

Rest active scan

Concentration active scan

Increased basal ganglia and deep limbic activity, seen on both studies.

with his performance. His wife started to relax around Robert because he appeared more present and loving toward her. In addition, Robert started an exercise program, ate more protein, and learned negative-thought-killing techniques.

Type 7, Unfocused Anxiety/Depression is best treated with stimulating antidepressants, such as Wellbutrin. Sometimes the use of stimulant medication is also added. Intense aerobic exercise is also helpful, as is a high-protein, low-carbohydrate diet.

A variant of Unfocused Anxiety/Depression is caused by overall reduced blood flow and activity to the cerebral cortex, in addition to too much activity in the basal ganglia and/or deep limbic system. The scan looks cold and dim and lacks appropriate activity, except in the emotional centers of the brain. This is a very striking finding. This pattern may be related to a number of factors, such as physical illness, drug or alcohol abuse, hypoxia (lack of oxygen), infectious agents, brain trauma, or exposure to toxic substances. This variant is often treatment resistant. Symptoms of this type include those listed above, plus frequent feelings of being sick, mental dullness, or cognitive impairment. In treating this variant it is important to explore for and eradicate the offending agents if possible. Here is an example:

Judy, the wife of a close friend, came to see us for problems with depression. She complained of a pervasive feeling of sadness, low energy, negativity, and difficulty concentrating. She was unable to care for her family as she desired. Her SPECT series showed overall markedly decreased activity, with the scalloping effect that is often associated with toxic exposure. She had no history of drug abuse or brain trauma. We recommended a medical workup to look for other physical causes of depression. We discovered she was severely anemic and had a very low red blood cell count. It was discovered that her anemia was caused by a vitamin B-12 deficiency. Correcting this problem was all it took to get Judy back on track.

It is important to note that some people may find that their symptoms do not fit neatly into any one type, that they have symptoms that seem to overlap several types or that they have suffered from more than one type of anxiety and/or depression in their life. When people have symptoms of more than one type, it is important to know which symptoms to treat first. We always treat Cyclic Anxiety/Depression and Temporal Lobe Anxiety/

Judy's SPECT Study, Before and After Vitamin B-12
(note overall improvement with treatment)

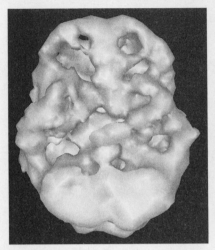

Before
Underside surface study
Overall decreased activity.

Before
Top-down surface study
Overall decreased activity.

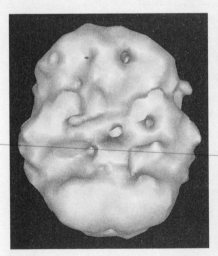

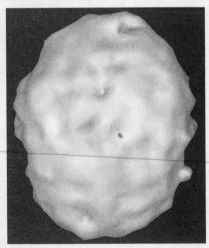

After
Underside surface study
Overall improved activity.

After
Top-down surface study
Overall improved activity.

Depression symptoms first. By treating these types first by using antiseizure medications, we believe we protect against many serious negative reactions to medication.

We hope you now have a sense of which type of anxiety/depression you or someone you love has and an idea of how to start doing something about it. The remainder of the book gives you more specific details and techniques for conquering these problems.

CHAPTER 5

Bio-Psycho-Social Assessment
of the Seven Types

nderstanding the story of a person's life and asking the right questions is the most important first step in the proper assessment of anxiety and depressive disorders and in the determination of the most accurate treatment and healing protocols. Although we have pioneered the use of brain SPECT imaging, which is extremely helpful in the diagnostic process, clinical history is the most important first step. While we use other tools—such as our checklists, SPECT studies, information from collateral sources such as spouses, and blood work—we find that a good clinical history is essential to proper diagnosis. It is most helpful to take a biological, psychological, and sociological approach when evaluating anxiety and depression. Evaluating problems in these three spheres increases the likelihood of obtaining the best possible evaluation and sets the stage for proper treatment.

Bio-Psycho-Social Assessment of Anxiety and Depression

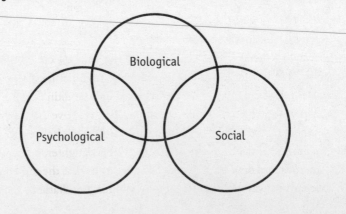

Biological Factors

Genetics

Because anxiety and depressive disorders run in families, family history is an important key to understanding a person's biology. When first talking to a patient we ask questions about grandparents from both sides and learn as much as possible about the parents, aunts, uncles, siblings, and children on each side. In the near future we may have DNA tests that look at our own genetic vulnerabilities.

From our clinical experience as well as a review of the medical literature, it seems that a very high percentage of anxiety and depressive disorders are passed down genetically. In our experience, if one parent has an anxiety or depressive disorder, 50 percent of the offspring will have one as well. If both parents have an anxiety or depressive disorder, 75 to 85 percent of the children will also be affected. We believe this familial predisposition contributes to the high incidence of family dysfunction when anxiety or depressive disorders are present.

A family came to see us from Israel with their ten-year-old son who had extreme problems with anxiety and depression. He was also oppositional, inflexible, and very stubborn. He had been refusing to go to school, and, overwhelmed with various fears, he slept on the floor of his parents' room. His SPECT study showed marked increased anterior cingulate gyrus activity and we determined he had Overfocused Anxiety/Depression. When we asked about the family history, the parents initially said no one else had these problems. However, when we described in detail the anterior cingulate gyrus and its function, the mother looked astonished. She said that her father had been the classic anterior cingulate personality. Although he didn't suffer from anxiety or depression, he was rigid, stubborn, had to have his way, and tormented others in the family with his selfish nature. He held grudges against family members for decades and, according to his daughter, made other people feel anxious and depressed. It seemed clear to us that the same underlying brain mechanism was working in the boy and his grandfather.

Medical Problems or Medications That
Can Mimic Anxiety and Depression

An overactive thyroid gland may cause symptoms that at first glance are almost indistinguishable from Type 1, Pure Anxiety, while an underactive thyroid might produce Type 2, Pure Depression–like or Type 7, Unfocused Anxiety/Depression–like symptoms. Likewise, medications such as asthma medications can make people look and feel anxious and some blood pressure medications can make people feel depressed. It is important for your doctor to assess the impact of medical problems on behavior. The following list of common medical problems associated with anxiety and depressive disorders is not exhaustive by any means, but highlights the correlation between physical health and "mental illness":

- Adrenal disease

- Anemia

- Brain injury

- Caffeine

- Caffeine withdrawal

- Cancer, especially pancreatic cancer

- Chronic Fatigue Syndrome (CFS)

- Hearing loss, often associated with social isolation and paranoia

- Infections or post-infectious states, such as post-pneumonia depression

- Low blood sugar states

- Migraines

- Mineral imbalances (copper excess/zinc deficiency)

- Mitral Valve Prolapse, seen in a higher percentage of anxious patients

- Pheochromocytoma (a rare tumor that produces excessive adrenaline)

- Syphilis or HIV

- Temporal Lobe Epilepsy

- Thyroid disease

- Vitamin deficiencies (especially thiamine, vitamin B-12, niacin)

- Many medications, such as birth control pills, weight loss pills, blood pressure medications, Accutane, even some antidepressants and tranquilizers

A battery of tests for new-onset anxiety or depression usually includes:

- Thyroid function—to rule out thyroid disease

- Complete blood count—to rule out anemia

- Urinalysis

- Urine drug screen—patients don't always tell us the truth about drug abuse

- Blood chemistry panel—to evaluate liver and kidney function, fasting blood sugar levels, electrolytes, among other things

- Zinc and copper levels

- HIV and syphilis screens

- Electrocardiogram

- Other tests as indicated by the history or examination

Brain Injury

Anxiety and depression often accompany brain injury. One of the most important lessons we've learned through our brain imaging work is that brain injuries can be very significant yet are often overlooked. Even "mild" brain injuries have a greater effect than most people, including physicians, realize. Brain SPECT imaging is often able to show areas of damage that are not seen on the anatomical studies like CT scans and MRI studies. We can see contra-coup injuries (opposite parts of the brain damaged by the same injury) and old injuries (even damage from birth or forcep deliveries). Brain injuries occur because of the structure of the brain and skull.

- Your brain is very soft. It is similar in consistency to soft butter or custard. It is easily bruised or damaged.

- Your skull is very hard. Inside your skull are many ridges, rough areas, and sharp, bony ridges.

- Your brain is in a closed space. When you experience a blow to the head there is no place for the brain to go, so it slams against the walls, ridges, and sharp, bony edges in the skull, ripping small blood vessels, causing micro-hemorrhaging (bleeding), and over time small areas of scar tissue form.

You do not have to lose consciousness in order to have a significant brain injury. Consciousness is controlled by structures deep in the brainstem. It is possible to have a significant injury to the cortex or surface of the brain, sparing the brainstem, and experience no loss of consciousness.

Concussions occur when the head either accelerates rapidly and then is stopped, or is spun rapidly. Violent shaking causes the brain cells to undergo metabolic changes. The damaged brain cells fire all their neurotransmitters at once in an unhealthy cascade, flooding the brain with chemicals, deadening certain receptors linked to learning and memory, and disrupting the cells' ability to transmit signals. While often there are no immediate symptoms and nothing irregular shows up on the CT scans or the MRI, subtle changes occur. Over a period of a few weeks or months, the individual may become tearful, angry, or irritable, and may have trouble thinking clearly or concentrating, or may suffer from headaches, confusion, blurred vision, memory loss, nausea, and sometimes unconsciousness. Other devastating symptoms can develop slowly over time. There may be personality changes, temper problems, dark thoughts, or difficulty expressing emotions or understanding others.

The brain areas especially vulnerable to injury include:

- temporal lobes, which house memory, receptive language, temper control, and mood stability;

- deep limbic system, which can cause problems with depression, negativity, and libido;

- prefrontal cortex, where judgment, concentration, attention span, impulse control, organization, planning, and expressive language are centered;

- anterior cingulate gyrus, the brain's gear shifter, where damage causes people to get stuck on negative thoughts or behaviors;

- parietal lobes, at the top–back part of the brain, coordinate and interpret sensory information from the opposite side of the body; they also handle directions, construction, and advanced mathematics; and

- occipital lobes, which can cause problems with visual processing.

Brain injuries can interrupt, delay, or alter social and intellectual development. In both children and adults, traumatic brain injuries can cause physical difficulties such as severe headaches, dizziness, fatigue, diminished

Three Examples of Brain Injuries Associated with Anxiety and Depression

15-year-old's brain injury from bicycle accident

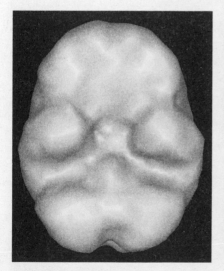 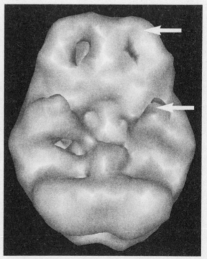

Normal underside surface view
Full, symmetrical activity.

Post-injury underside surface view
Notice flattening of the prefront cortex (top arrow) and decreased left and right anterior temporal lobe activity (lower arrow).

motor skills, and other problems. They also can create mental difficulties such as memory loss, difficulty with concentration, depression, hypersensitivity to noise, photophobia (hypersensitivity to light), and so on. Often the most challenging problems for families are the emotional and social difficulties that may arise after a traumatic brain injury, such as increased incidence of psychiatric problems, which are common after traumatic brain injury, even when the injury is relatively mild. A high percentage of those suffering even a mild concussion experience depression within the first two years following the injury. In addition, those with mild concussions experience an increased incidence of substance abuse, marital problems, job-related problems, as well as incarceration and other legal problems.

A number of years ago Dr. Amen wrote a newspaper article on brain injuries. On the day the article appeared in the paper, Dr. Amen received a call from a distraught mother. Four years earlier her sixteen-year-old son had sustained a brain injury from a bicycle accident when the front tire of his bi-

35-year-old's brain injury from skiing accident

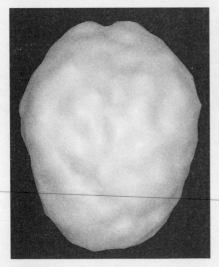 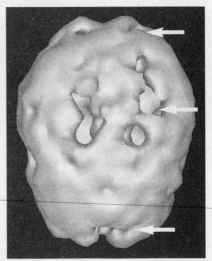

Normal top-down surface view
Full, symmetrical activity.

Post-injury top-down surface view
Notice decreased prefrontal cortex pole (bottom arrow), decreased parietal lobes (middle arrow), and decreased occipital lobes (top arrow).

cycle hit a curb and he flipped over the handlebars and landed on the left side of his face. He was unconscious for about thirty minutes. Over the next several months his personality changed dramatically. He went from being a straight-A student and a sweet young man to someone who had no interest in school and was easily angered and depressed. He also started drinking alcohol on a regular basis. Three years after the injury he shot and killed himself. His mother had blamed herself for his downward spiral. Fortunately Dr. Amen's article helped her understand the terrible tragedy. No one had told her the negative impact a brain injury can have. Likely, her son had injured his left temporal lobe and prefrontal cortex, causing him to have problems with aggressive behavior toward himself, judgment, and impulse control.

Unrecognized brain injuries often trigger anxiety or depressive disorders. In fact, people with brain injuries have a threefold increase in anxiety and depressive disorders. Brain injuries tend to cluster in Types 6 and 7 anxiety and depression, as they tend to affect the temporal and frontal lobes. Damage to the frontal lobes can disinhibit the deep limbic system and make a person more likely to feel sad, negative, and emotionally overwhelmed. Studying World War II veterans with and without significant brain injuries, Dr. Tracey

52-year-old's brain injury from motor vehicle accident

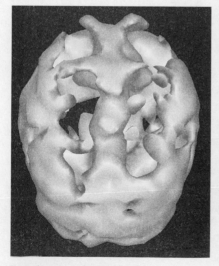 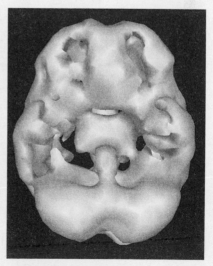

Top-down surface view
Marked decreased prefrontal
and temporal lobes.

Underside surface view
Marked decreased parietal and
occipital lobes.

Holsinger and colleagues at Duke University confirmed the connection between brain injury and depression, concluding that brain injuries significantly increase the risk for depression up to fifty years after the initial injury.

It is interesting to note that many people forget that they have had significant brain injuries. Typically we ask patients five times during the course of their examination whether or not they have had a significant brain injury. Many people say no, over and over again, and then "all of a sudden" remember a significant fall, car accident, or other trauma.

Frank, forty-two, came to see us for problems with depression and concentration. His scan showed a big dent in his left prefrontal cortex and temporal lobes consistent with a brain injury. When asked about falls, car accidents, or fights, he responded no. Finally, when we asked him if he played sports, he said, "Yes. I played football for San Francisco City High School."

"Ever get your bell rung?" we asked.

An astonished look came over Frank. He said, "Why, yes. I completely forgot. We had this crazy coach who used to pair us up and we had to get twenty yards apart. He would make us bend down and run at each other full speed headfirst and bang helmets together. One time after we did that I was dizzy for three weeks and had trouble learning in school."

Chronic Fatigue Syndrome (CFS)

Many doctors have dismissed patients who complain of Chronic Fatigue Syndrome as crocks, or have written them off as having "personality" problems. Our scans have taught us that CFS is often the result of some toxic insult to the brain and shows patterns similar to a brain infection or encephalitis. We classically see hyperactivity in the limbic brain and overall decreased activity.

Toxic Exposure

When the brain is exposed to toxic substances it is much more likely to show symptoms of emotional problems. Brain infections such as meningitis and encephalitis cause toxic inflammation in the brain and damage tissue. Clearly, fetal exposure to drugs, alcohol, and cigarettes also puts a child at risk for problems. Often mothers who use these substances during pregnancy are medicating their own struggles with depression or anxiety. The

Chronic Fatigue Syndrome Scan

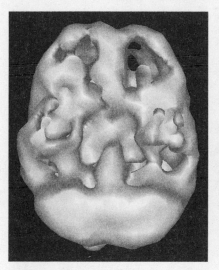 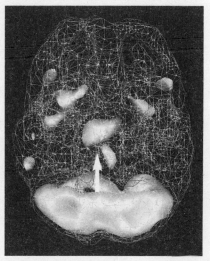

Underside surface view
Severe overall decreased activity.

Underside active view
Increased deep limbic activity (arrow).

baby not only inherits a predisposition to these problems, but he experiences toxicity to his brain. Environmental toxins can also have a seriously negative effect on brain function and cause anxiety and depressive symptoms.

Roger and Mary Ann came to see us at the request of their marital therapist. Roger had a problem with his temper, and he felt chronically nervous and uptight and frequently thought about suicide. We diagnosed him with Type 6, Temporal Lobe Anxiety/Depression and felt he may have temporal lobe problems. He had no history of head trauma or illegal drug abuse. His SPECT study showed marked overall scalloping and decreased activity in his left temporal lobe as well as increased basal ganglia and deep limbic activity. His scan clearly showed a toxic effect. Roger worked in a furniture factory in an area with poor ventilation so he was frequently exposed to high concentrations of toxic fumes from the finishing varnishes. In addition to medication and psychotherapy, it was essential for Roger to get better ventilation and avoid exposure to high levels of toxic fumes. Sometimes just eliminating the toxic substances is enough to promote healing.

Roger's Toxic Exposure Scan

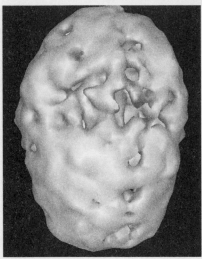

Top-down surface view
Overall decreased activity with
scalloping.

Underside surface view
Overall decreased activity with
scalloping.

Drug Abuse

It is important to screen for drug abuse when assessing for anxiety and depression or any other psychiatric disorder because anxiety, depression, and
drug abuse very commonly occur together. Drug abuse itself may masquerade
as either anxiety or depression. Because many drug abusers are not honest during the interview (because of shame or fear of being found out), we often order a drug screen to rule out our suspicions even if they have denied taking
drugs. While drug screens are not foolproof, we have found that just the act of
ordering the screen is revealing. If we say, "I want to order a drug screen. I
know you said you aren't using drugs, but people who use drugs often won't
admit it. I just want to do a thorough evaluation and make sure" and the person responds, "I don't believe in drug screens. They are not reliable. I won't do
it," it is generally a good indicator that he is using drugs. If he says, "No problem, I understand," and willingly submits to the test, it is generally a sign that
he is not using drugs. Of course, we have been fooled, so even if a patient
agrees, we send the specimen to the lab if we are at all suspicious.

Ecstasy Scan vs Normal

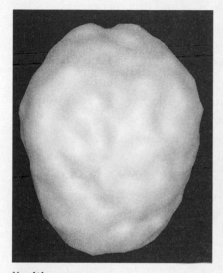 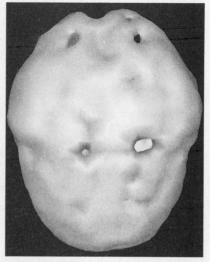

Healthy scan
Top-down surface view
Full, even, symmetrical activity.

Ecstasy scan
Top-down surface view
Scalloping noted.

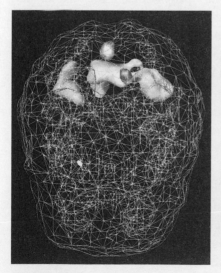 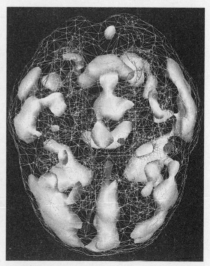

Healthy scan
Top-down active view
Good activity in the cerebellum;
cool everywhere else.

Ecstasy scan
Top-down surface view
Marked increased anterior cingulate,
basal ganglia, and deep limbic activity.

Drug and alcohol abuse is commonly used to unconsciously self-medicate anxiety and depression. In our experience, alcohol, heroin, and marijuana use are common in Types 1 through 5 to settle internal pain, anxiety, sadness, and restlessness, while cocaine and methamphetamines are used to feel more energetic and focused (types 5 through 7). Nicotine use (cigarettes, cigars, and chewing tobacco) is more common in people with Type 7, as is the use of large amounts of caffeine. Nicotine and caffeine are mild stimulants.

Substance abuse, while seeming to be an effective temporary solution, often makes anxiety and depressive symptoms much worse over time. Brain imaging work has clearly taught us how harmful drug abuse is to brain function. Cocaine, methamphetamines, alcohol, marijuana, nicotine, and caffeine decrease brain activity over time, sometimes significantly. One study by Dr. Ismael Mena at UCLA showed that cocaine addicts had, overall, 23 percent less brain activity compared to a group of people who had never used drugs. The cocaine addicts in the study who smoked had 45 percent less activity in their brains. The smokers did not have access to nearly half of their brains. Ecstasy is also damaging to the brain. Many people with depression abuse ecstasy because, in the short run, it makes them feel better by aiding in the release of the neurotransmitter serotonin. Unfortunately, it depletes serotonin stores in the brain and makes people look more anxious, depressed, and obsessive over time. Dr. Amen was involved with an *America Undercover* HBO special on ecstasy, and he scanned a nineteen-year-old man who had used it heavily over the prior year. The young man's brain manifested severe Obsessive-Compulsive Disorder with flaming hot activity in his anterior cingulate gyrus and basal ganglia. It was literally one of the hottest (most overactive) brains Dr. Amen had ever seen.

SAMANTHA

Samantha, a twenty-two-year-old college senior, came to us for help for severe anxiety. She often felt isolated and alone, and she was having trouble finishing her degree because she would not take the required speech and communication classes for fear of speaking in public. She said, "I would rather take an F in a class than suffer through the anxiety of thinking about giving a speech or even talking in class." Samantha drank heavily on the weekends and said it was the only time she felt calm and was able to socialize. As part of her evaluation we ordered a brain SPECT study, which showed marked increased basal ganglia activity (as in Type 1, Pure Anxiety) and overall scalloping, an indication of damage from her alcohol use. Seeing the alcohol-caused damage on her scan convinced Samantha to stop drinking. We treated her with biofeedback, supplements, and therapy. Within three months she was able to take and pass her speech class, and she felt more relaxed, overall, without alcohol.

AMIR

Amir, a thirty-five-year-old computer technician, had suffered from depression for as long as he could remember. He even looked sad in his childhood pictures. At the age of thirty he had a skiing accident that tore the ligaments in his right knee. After knee surgery his surgeon put him on a common opiate painkiller, hydrocodone. Amir found that not only did the painkiller help his post-surgical knee pain but also dramatically eased his depression. He felt happier, more positive, and more social. He liked the painkiller so much that he took the entire bottle in half the allotted time. At first his surgeon refilled the prescription early without question, but at the second request he insisted that Amir come in for "a chat." It was clear to the surgeon

Amir's Scan

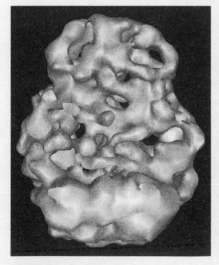 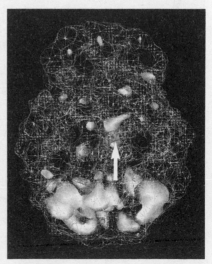

Underside surface view
Severe overall decreased activity with scalloping (bumpiness).

Underside active view
Increased deep limbic activity (arrow).

that Amir was becoming dependent on and abusing the hydrocodone, and he refused to renew the prescription. Amir went doctor shopping and found several doctors who would prescribe it for him. After a year of using more and more hydrocodone, a pharmacist got suspicious that he was abusing the medication because his prescriptions were from several different physicians. The pharmacist notified all of Amir's known treating doctors, and his primary physician referred Amir to an addiction specialist. The addiction specialist, having seen this pattern many times before, sent Amir to our clinic for a psychiatric evaluation. His scans revealed Type 2, Pure Depression, but also drug damage from his excessive hydrocodone abuse. Hydrocodone works very much like heroin in the brain and often causes severely decreased blood flow to the brain. It was clear from the scan and his history that Amir was self-medicating his depression, but with a very toxic substance. Through drug treatment and treatment for his depression, Amir was able to heal and feel better than he had felt at any time in his life. The pharmacist saved Amir's brain and ultimately his life.

JEREMY

Seventeen-year-old Jeremy was failing in school. He refused to do his homework, often skipped class, and on several occasions his parents found him intoxicated and high on marijuana. He isolated himself in his room, spent little time with friends, and withdrew into himself. Additionally, he seemed anxious and nervous and often complained of stomachaches and headaches. The change in his behavior seemed to be triggered by a family move during the middle of tenth grade. On the recommendation of Jeremy's school counselor, his parents brought him in for evaluation. Through our interview with his parents, we discovered a family history of depression and anxiety. Jeremy's SPECT scan showed markedly increased activity in the basal ganglia, deep limbic areas, and anterior cingulate gyrus, as well as scalloping across the cortical surface (likely the toxic effect from substance abuse). Jeremy was seen by a psychotherapist, put on an antidepressant, and given random drug testing. As the depression and anxiety lifted, his desire to use drugs lessened and he was able to do better in school and at home.

Jeremy's Scan

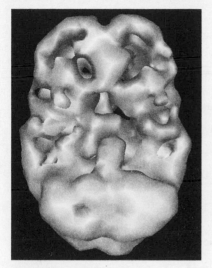

Underside surface view
Severe overall decreased activity
with scalloping (bumpiness).

Underside active view
Increased basal ganglia (middle arrow),
deep limbic (bottom arrow) and
anterior cingulate gyrus activity
(top arrow).

Hormonal Influences

Hormonal influences play a major role in anxiety and depression, especially in women. The incidence of depressive disorders in boys and girls is roughly equivalent, but after girls enter puberty, the incidence of depression doubles. Anxiety and depressive symptoms also tend to be exacerbated in the premenstrual period, after a woman has a baby, and around the time of menopause. A number of SPECT studies have shown overall decreased brain activity with decreased estrogen levels. During perimenopause or menopause, many women experience problems with energy. Estrogen replacement, although controversial, appears to have a positive effect on brain function. Fluctuating hormonal levels clearly impact how the brain works, including seizure frequency and intensity. Estrogen and progesterone, which regulate ovarian function, also affect the excitability of neurons in the cerebral cortex. Either hormone can occupy receptor sites for GABA—a widespread inhibitory neurotransmitter. When estrogen occupies these receptors, it has a proconvulsant effect and may cause an area to be more active, putting a woman at greater risk for anxiety or depression. Progesterone's effects are directly opposite. When progesterone occupies the GABA receptors, it tends to suppress activity and leads to a net anticonvulsant effect. In this way, for females with epilepsy or mood and anxiety disorders, changes in the balance of sex hormones throughout their lives may alter the frequency and intensity of brain function, seizures, and their moods. We ask women where they are in their menstrual cycle because it may have an impact on their scan findings.

Psychological Factors

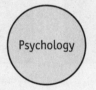

Early Neglect and Abuse

Both physical and emotional neglect and abuse play a role in anxiety and depression because the brain needs nurturing and appropriate stimulation to develop properly. An extreme example of neglect occurred during the late 1980s when thousands of Romanian orphans were raised without affection, touching, or nurturing. Many of these children developed severe emotional, learning, and behavioral problems and subsequent scans showed overall decreased activity in their brains. Without appropriate stimulation, connections between neurons in the brain are not created. Emotional or physical abuse causes a rush of stress hormones and chemicals that can poison a baby or child's brain. Additionally stress hormones in animals have been found to damage the memory centers. Chronic stress also causes the brain to reset itself and become hyperalert, which can lead to severe anxiety and mood swings.

Negative Self-Talk

Low self-esteem, self-doubt, and a lack of confidence can stem from negative thinking patterns. Most of us are never taught how to think. We have classes on reading, math, English, and history, but rarely are there classes on the most basic of all cognitive functions—how to think in clear, logical, and helpful ways. Of course, having anxiety or depressive illnesses makes one more prone to negative thought patterns, but these negative thought patterns can also cause negative brain changes. Negative self-talk can result from living in a chronically negative environment, although this is not always the case. Correcting negative thought patterns with therapy is an essential step in healing.

Learned Helplessness

"Learned helplessness" is a concept that originated in experiments with dogs many years ago. In the first part of the experiment, a group of dogs were exposed to electric shocks but were able to stop the shocks by pressing a panel. A second group of dogs were exposed to shocks but were unable to stop the shocks. When the first group of dogs were later exposed to a different kind of electric shock situation, they rapidly learned that they could escape the shocks by jumping over a barrier. But when the second group of dogs were exposed to the new situation, they made no attempt to escape. Instead, they whimpered and sat down. The second group of dogs had "learned that the situation was hopeless" and they displayed "learned helplessness."

Psychologist Martin Seligman used the term "learned helplessness" to describe his observations of depressed patients. We have also seen this phenomenon again and again in both anxious and depressed patients. Learned helplessness occurs when a person tries repeatedly to be successful in school or relationships or other important areas of life but performs poorly. Demoralized, she gives up. The demoralization contributes heavily to anxiety and depressive symptoms.

Through the years the concept of learned helplessness has been studied as it relates to human behavior, especially with depressed patients. The negative self-talk that is commonly present with patients who have anxiety and depression, the self-doubt, the loss of self-esteem, and the tendency to look for evidence of failure and dwell on it are all-too-familiar issues for any therapist working with this population. Not all of these complaints resolve with medication management alone, even when the other symptoms of anxiety and depression improve. Because medication can't eliminate negative self-talk, we strongly encourage cognitive-behavioral therapeutic interventions and other supportive therapies in addition to medication.

Social and Societal Factors

Sociology

Social Situation

In order to get a full picture of a patient's life, doctors and mental health professionals ask questions about everything from relationships to employment, family history of mental illness to physical, emotional, and sexual abuse patterns in the family, recent changes—positive or negative—in the patient's life to drug and alcohol use. This information is of vital importance because these factors may affect both the development and the outcome of the patient's illness. Conversely, the patient's illness may affect or produce disturbance within his or her social and family system.

Societal Contributions to Anxiety and Depressive Disorders

Anxiety and depression are diagnosed more today compared to generations past. Improved symptom recognition, even when combined with decreased stigma associated with mental illness, is not enough to explain the increase.

Our society is more mobile than it was a generation or two ago. People no longer live and work in the same community in which they were born and raised, which disrupts family and friendships. Military families can generally expect to make many relocations; others can expect to make several moves in their lifetime because of job needs or education requirements. Adding to the disruption of family ties is the high rate of divorce in modern society and the all-too-common emotional and financial abandonment of women and children.

Rates of addiction have escalated. The rates of alcoholism and drug and nicotine abuse continue to rise, becoming one of the greatest problems facing our society today. Fetal exposure to these substances is a primary health care concern because of the lifelong consequences for the child. However, people abuse themselves in many ways and are addicted to substances besides alcohol and drugs. The rate of childhood obesity is a national health care crisis, and as many as 50 percent of adults in America are overweight. Additionally, we are addicted to negative self-talk and a self-centered lifestyle.

The rate of depression and anxiety has increased more for women than for men because of the unique social, economic, and biological pressures facing women. Most women need to work to help support their family, whether they are in a committed relationship or single, yet they earn far less than men even when performing the same tasks. On average, working mothers who are married still perform 89 percent of housework and 78 percent of child care duties, according to most studies and surveys. Women are tired and also have to contend with hormonal transitions that are risk factors for triggering anxiety and depression.

Finally, living with or caring for elderly parents is becoming more common as the baby boomer generation ages. At the same time, this generation is also caring for their children, which can be overwhelming. Caregivers are frequently at risk for depression and stress–related symptoms such as headaches and muscle aches. Living with family members who are ill or who have psychiatric illnesses are also risk factors for causing symptoms in other family members.

No one lives in a vacuum, and obtaining a full bio-psycho-social evaluation is the best way to ensure proper diagnosis and treatment.

CHAPTER 6

Effective Treatment for
the Seven Types

The Amen Clinic Brain/Life Enhancement Program is geared toward optimizing both brain and life function for all patients. Medication is commonly the only treatment prescribed for anxiety and depression, but is rarely effective as a sole intervention. We have developed a holistic approach to treatment because elimination of all symptoms is our goal. The Amen Clinic Brain/Life Enhancement Program includes treatment plans for each type of depression and anxiety that incorporate education and therapy and support recommendations, dietary suggestions, fitness plans, supplements, medications, and specific behavioral interventions. We believe "people need skills not just pills" to optimize brain and life function.

While not everyone will need all the Amen Clinic Brain/Life Enhancement Program interventions suggested for their type of anxiety and depression, we have found that patients achieve the best results by incorporating a variety of them. Because anxiety and depression have clear biological roots, and serious psychological and social consequences when left untreated, these causes and ramifications respond to precise interventions.

We often use the following computer analogy with our patients: In order for a computer to run a program effectively, its hardware must be sufficient. It must have enough RAM, disk space, and processing speed. Trying to run complex programs, such as Microsoft Excel, on an old 286 computer with only 4 megabytes of RAM just won't work. Yet many people with anxiety and/or depression do not have enough RAM (short-term memory), disk space, or processing speed in their brains because of underactivity in their prefrontal cortex and temporal lobes. Others get stuck in loops of thought because of anterior cingulate gyrus hyperactivity. To run programs effectively you must first optimize the hardware—the brain. Once a computer's hardware is optimized, it still has programming needs. Because of the hardware (brain) problems, many people with anxiety and/or depression have trouble utilizing psychotherapy, a software program. Once the brain is optimized, it is important to input strategies that help people with anxiety and/or depression to be more effective in their daily lives.

Assessing anxiety and depression within the bio–psycho–social model is important. Treatment applied within this context is fundamental to achieving the best possible integration of a person's brain (biology), mind-set (psychology), and functioning within relationships (sociology). Neglecting any of these areas leaves a person vulnerable and can lead to treatment failure.

Effective Bio-psycho-social Interventions for the Seven Types

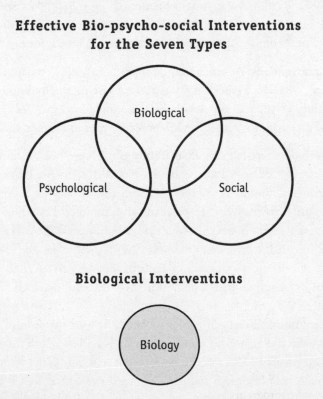

Biological Interventions

Eliminate anything toxic: Toxic substances can cause as well as exacerbate anxiety and depressive symptoms (for example, marijuana use can make someone appear as though he has Type 7, Unfocused Anxiety/Depression). Drug abuse treatment is often very important in healing anxiety/depression.

Caffeine and nicotine have been shown in brain studies to decrease overall blood flow to the brain, which in turn makes it harder to treat anxiety and depressive disorders. In addition, in our experience both nicotine and caffeine decrease the effectiveness of medication and supplement treatments and increase the number of side effects people experience. In the short run caffeine may make you feel more focused; unfortunately, it also decreases brain blood flow and over time can make it more difficult to heal. Other toxic substances to avoid or eliminate may be revealed by a blood screen. Any medications that contribute to anxiety and depression must be stopped as well.

Protect your head: Head injuries can take a mild case of anxiety or depression and add temporal lobe dysfunction. It is critical to prevent head injuries if possible. Kids should always wear helmets when riding bikes, snowboarding, or Rollerblading, and they should not hit soccer balls with their heads. Seat belts are essential. Avoid activities that put you at risk for head injuries.

Dietary interventions: As our colleague Barry Sears, Ph.D. (coauthor of *The Zone*), says, "Food is a powerful drug. You can use it to help mood and cognitive ability or you can unknowingly make things worse." We explore dietary interventions for anxiety and depressive types in chapter 9.

Intense aerobic exercise and weight training: All types benefit from intense aerobic exercise because exercise boosts blood flow to the brain. Exercise also increases serotonin availability in the brain, which has a tendency to calm cingulate hyperactivity. Tryptophan, the amino acid building block for serotonin, is a relatively small molecule. It does not compete well against the larger amino acids to cross into the brain. With intense aerobic exercise the large muscles use the bigger amino acids to replenish tissue. This decreases competition for tryptophan, which ultimately leads to increased concentrations within the brain.

We recommend that our patients exercise at least five times a week for thirty to forty-five minutes. Often, a fast walk is sufficient, but the heart rate must be elevated. We also recommend weight training. Active weight training can raise your heart rate and increases your strength as well as your self-esteem.

Medication: Medication is an emotionally loaded issue for many people. There is a lot of controversy in this area. After doing brain imaging work for the past thirteen years, it is clear that medication can be very helpful for many patients, and withholding it from some patients is downright neglectful. Medication is one of the best-studied and most effective treatments for anxiety and depressive disorders. However, medication by itself is generally bad treatment and can make some people worse. Unfortunately, most people neglect the psychological and social aspects of anxiety and depression and take medication only. Medication for each type is discussed in chapter 7.

Supplements: Even more controversial than medication is using natural supplements for anxiety or depressive disorders. There is conflicting research behind using supplements with anxiety and depressive disorders, but what there is indicates that supplements can be useful for mild to moderate conditions. Our clinical experience has shown that supplements can be helpful when used in a thoughtful way. Our worry is that people spend billions of dollars on these treatments with little regard to effectiveness or side effects. Because supplements are "natural," people think of them as innocuous, which isn't true in our experience. While we are not opposed to natural supplements (we often recommend them), we are opposed to a person being treated ineffectively. A rational, balanced approach to both medication and supplement treatment is needed. Supplement treatment for anxiety and depressive types is discussed in chapter 8.

Psychological Interventions

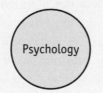

Education

Education about anxiety and depressive disorders, their impact on home, school, family, and the self, is the first step in treatment. Robert Pasnau, M.D., past president of the American Psychiatric Association, said that coping requires three things: information, self-esteem, and a sense of control. Obtaining accurate information is the critical first step in treating anxiety and depression. The more accurate information you have, the more likely you are to get the best help.

Correcting automatic negative thoughts: Negativity is one of the hallmarks of anxiety and depressive disorders. Excessive negative thoughts predispose a person to anxiety and depression. In chapter 10, we teach you how to identify and rid yourself of negative thoughts (we call them ANTs—automatic negative thoughts) that invade your life.

Targeted psychotherapy: For many people with anxiety or depressive disorders there are a number of psychological issues that need to be addressed. Without the proper biological treatment, psychotherapy can be a fruitless and frustrating experience for both the therapist and the patient. We have consulted with many anxious and depressed patients who have been in psychotherapy for years without much benefit. For many, when they were placed on the right medication or supplements, dramatic improvement occurred in several weeks. This is not to say that psychotherapy is not a necessary component of treatment, but it often needs to be done in combination with the right biological treatment, as anxiety and depressive disorders have strong neuro-biological underpinnings.

Eye Movement Desensitization and Reprocessing (EMDR)

Eye Movement Desensitization and Reprocessing (EMDR) is a powerful tool to counteract anxiety and help heal painful past memories. The focus of EMDR is the resolution of emotional distress arising from difficult childhood memories, or the recovery from traumatic events such as automobile accidents, assaults, natural disasters, and combat trauma. EMDR was developed by psychologist Francine Shapiro in 1987. While walking around a lake she noticed that a disturbing thought disappeared when her eyes spontaneously started to move back and forth from the lower left to the upper right visual fields. She tried it again with another anxiety-provoking thought and found that the anxious feeling went away. In the days that followed she tried the technique with friends, acquaintances, and interested students and found the technique helpful in relieving anxiety. She then went further to work with patients and developed a technique that is now used worldwide.

The mainstay of the EMDR technique involves having clients bring up emotionally troubling memories while their eyes follow a trained therapist's hand moving horizontally back and forth. Following a specific protocol, the clinician helps the client identify the images, negative beliefs, emotions, and body sensations associated with a targeted memory or event. Through the therapy, positive statements and beliefs replace negative ones. The believability of this new thought is rated while the client thinks of the disturbing event. The goal of EMDR treatment is the rapid processing of information about the negative experience and movement toward an adaptive resolution. This means a reduction in the client's distress, a shift in the client's negative belief to positive belief, and the possibility of more optimal behavior in relationships and at work.

EMDR is one of the most rapid and effective treatments we have ever personally seen as psychiatrists. It is important that EMDR be done by a trained therapist. You can contact the EMDR International Association at *www.EMDRIA.org* for a list of certified EMDR therapists. According to EMDRIA, "No one knows for sure how EMDR works but through brain-imaging techniques we are beginning to see its effects." What research has suggested so far is that when a person is upset, the brain cannot process information in its usual manner. The event that provoked the upsetting feelings becomes "frozen in time," and "stuck" in the information-processing system (anterior cingulate gyrus). When a person remembers this event, he becomes flooded with the sights, sounds, smells, thoughts, and emotions of the original event as intensely as when it actually occurred. Such upsetting memories may have a profoundly negative impact on the way a person sees the world and relates to other people. Present-day incidents and interactions restimulate the experience of this upsetting event. EMDR appears to produce a direct effect on the way the brain processes upsetting material. Researchers have suggested that the eye movements trigger a neurophysiological mechanism that activates an accelerated information processing system. Accelerated information processing is a phrase used in EMDR to describe the rapid working through, 'metabolizing,' of upsetting experiences. Following successful EMDR treatment, the upsetting experiences are worked through to adaptive resolution. The person receiving EMDR comes to understand that the event is in the past, realizes appropriately who or what was responsible for the event, and feels more certain about present-day safety and the capacity to make choices. What happened can still be remembered by the person, but with much less upset.

An analysis of fifty-nine studies of PTSD treatments indicated that EMDR and behavior therapy were both effective for reducing the symptoms of PTSD. EMDR treatment time was shorter than behavior therapy (five versus fifteen hours). Other controlled studies have shown that EMDR is effective in treating phobias, in reducing stress in law-enforcement employees, and in helping reduce the distress experienced by traumatized children.

Under the guidance of psychologist Jennifer Lendl, an EMDR trainer, and Karen Lansing, MFCC, we have been recommending EMDR for the past seven years. We have seen it be very helpful for anxiety reduction, PTSD, and performance enhancement. We have studied EMDR with brain SPECT imaging before, during, and after treatment. EMDR changes brain function and calms the overactive focal areas of the brain. In PTSD, for example, we see a diamond pattern on SPECT, which indicates excessive activity in the anterior cingulate gyrus (top point of the diamond), basal ganglia (two side points of the diamond), and limbic-thalamus (bottom point of the diamond). People who have been traumatized and develop PTSD symptoms (such as flashbacks, nightmares, worries, quick startle, anxiety, depression, and avoidance) are frequently overly concerned and worried (anterior cingulate gyrus traits), anxious and hyperalert (basal ganglia), and they filter everything through negativity (deep limbic system). EMDR calms all of these areas on SPECT.

KRYSTLE

Krystle, thirty-two, was involved in a traffic accident when a truck veered across the center dividing line into her lane and she had to swerve off the road and landed in a ditch. For weeks she had problems sleeping, experienced constant anxiety, and couldn't drive. She cried a lot and often flashed back to the accident. She had no prior history of trauma. Her before-treatment SPECT study showed the diamond pattern: overactivity in the anterior cingulate gyrus, basal ganglia, and limbic areas. After three sessions with EMDR, Krystle felt significantly better, slept better, was less anxious, and was able to drive. When we repeated her SPECT study there was marked calming of activity in all three areas.

Focused breathing: One technique that we have found very helpful for our anxiety disorder patients is diaphragmatic breathing. This technique helps impulse control, temper outbursts, anxiety, and clarity of thought. It is discussed in chapter 12.

Krystle's: Before and After Treatment with EMDR

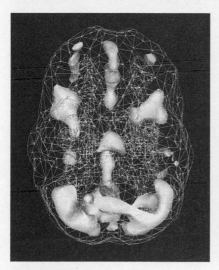 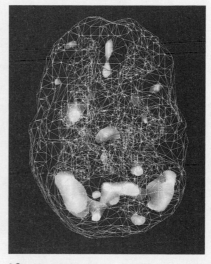

Before treatment
Increased anterior cingulate gyrus, BG, and DLS.

After treatment
Overall calming of the anterior cingulate gyrus, BG, and DLS.

Social Interventions

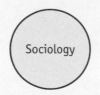

Sociology

Support

Obtaining support for yourself and your family is critical. Many people with anxiety or depressive disorders or who have it in their family feel isolated and alone. A sense of relief can come from knowing that other people have the same or a similar illness as you. In addition, interacting with other families with anxiety and depression can give you more ideas about coping strategies for specific situations. There are many ways to get emotional support for anxiety and depressive disorders.

There are many websites that offer support group sections for a wide variety of problems, including anxiety and depression. The Internet often provides the very latest information. Look under "anxiety" or "depression" in the search functions of these services. A word of caution about the Internet: Because anyone can write on the Internet, check out the information you obtain with your personal physician. One of us once treated a person who had obtained information on the Internet to use high doses of a cough syrup to treat his depression and trouble focusing. He became paranoid and angry, and he lost his job and his marriage because of his behavior on the drug. A list of helpful Internet sites is found at the end of this book.

A local community support group can be a source of great information. There are support groups for anxiety and depression all over the country. Look in your local paper or on Internet search engines to find a support group in your area.

Interpersonal strategies: Getting along with others is often difficult for people with anxiety and depression. In treating people of all ages with anxiety and depression, it is often important to include an interpersonal psychotherapy component in the treatment. Interpersonal psychotherapy is discussed in chapter 11.

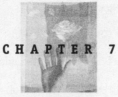

CHAPTER 7

Mindful Medication for
the Seven Types

When optimal brain and life function is the goal, medication is often an important component of effective treatment for the seven types of anxiety and depression. Because these disorders have strong neurobiological underpinnings, they need biological intervention. When symptoms are mild, biological therapies such as supplements, diet, exercise, and so on can replace the need for medication. At other times, medication can be lifesaving.

Whenever medication is started or considered, it is essential to have clear goals in mind for its use. Some examples of treatment goals include:

- improving mood and mood stability;

- calming anxiety, nervousness, fear, and panic;

- calming muscle tension and excessive motor output (such as nail biting, tics, and hair pulling);

- decreasing irritability;

- increasing motivation and interest in life;

- improving memory;

- improving sleep patterns and energy levels;

- improving flexibility;

- improving outlook and optimism;

- improving cognitive ability and clarity of thought;

- improving sexual desire;

- decreasing worrying, obsessive thoughts, and compulsive behaviors;

- eliminating suicidal thoughts and behaviors;

- improving overall functioning at school, at work, at home, in relationships, and individually.

Ideally your physician will cover these issues when prescribing medication, but the following are helpful guidelines:

- In almost all cases, start only one medication at a time. If you start more than one medicine at a time you will not know which one worked or which one caused any side effects.

- Write down exactly how to take your medication when you are in the doctor's office. Too many patients are confused about how to take their medication.

- Do exactly what the doctor says, as far as dose, timing of the medication, and how long you are supposed to take it. Too many patients play doctor and alter their dose without checking with a trained professional first. Also, ask what to do if you miss a dose.

- Keep a daily mood log or rating sheet to see how the medication or medications are working. We have our patients choose two, three, or four major symptoms and rate them on a scale of 1 to 10, where 1 is terrible and 10 is great. Our form follows.

- Do not try to get away with the least amount of medication possible. You want the best dose, not the least dose.

- Do not take medication with citrus juices, such as orange or grapefruit juice, as they tend to deactivate some medications.

- If your goal is to take less medication, make sure you exercise, eat the right diet, and do the appropriate therapy for your situation.

- Be organized for your follow-up sessions. Write down questions ahead of time. Be prepared to give a full assessment of how the medications are working.

The Amen Clinic Medication Dosing Instructions & Monthly Medication Rating Sheet

Name: _____ Date: _____

Medications: _____

Treatment Day	Dose	Time of Day			
		Morning	**Midday**	**Afternoon**	**Bedtime**

Please rate yourself or your child daily in the areas of mood (m), anxiety (a), and concentration (c) on a scale of 1 to 10 (1 = terrible, 10 = great)

Date	Dosage	m/a/c	Date	Dosage	m/a/c
_____	_____	_____	_____	_____	_____
_____	_____	_____	_____	_____	_____
_____	_____	_____	_____	_____	_____
_____	_____	_____	_____	_____	_____
_____	_____	_____	_____	_____	_____
_____	_____	_____	_____	_____	_____
_____	_____	_____	_____	_____	_____
_____	_____	_____	_____	_____	_____
_____	_____	_____	_____	_____	_____
_____	_____	_____	_____	_____	_____
_____	_____	_____	_____	_____	_____

Medication should be targeted to each type of anxiety and depression and tailored to each individual patient. Even the best medications can make things much worse if they are rendered ineffective through incorrect application. When treatments fail, individuals and families get discouraged. Discouragement leads people to stop treatment. While many physicians feel that it's OK to try treatments until they eventually get the right one, in our experience, a doctor has only three tries to get medication right for a patient—fewer if the patient dislikes the doctor. If a treatment plan is working, patients are much more willing to stick with it.

Type 1: Pure Anxiety—Hot Basal Ganglia (BG)

From a medication perspective, Type 1, Pure Anxiety, caused by an overflow of activity in the basal ganglia, is best treated by medications that calm the brain. The cautious use of benzodiazepines, buspirone, antidepressants (especially the tricyclic antidepressants desipramine and imipramine), and anticonvulsants are often effective in calming the focal hot areas in this part of the brain.

Benzodiazepines were previously some of the most commonly prescribed medications in the United States. Unfortunately, doctors other than psychiatrists often prescribed them indiscriminately. This led to widespread abuse, and in recent years physicians have become much more cautious about prescribing this class of drug. Benzodiazepines tend to be very effective and quick-acting anti-anxiety medications, especially when immediate relief from the symptoms of anxiety is necessary and when substance abuse is not a concern. However, they have several drawbacks, including the tendency to cause memory problems, tiredness, confusion, addiction, and a severe withdrawal syndrome if they are abruptly discontinued. On SPECT studies we often see overall markedly decreased brain activity from these medications. Benzodiazepines are also very dangerous when combined with alcohol or other sedating drugs. Xanax, Valium, and Klonopin are examples of commonly prescribed benzodiazepines.

One of the best uses of benzodiazepines is in the early stages of treatment of anxiety and/or depression when a tricyclic antidepressant or selective serotonin reuptake inhibitor has also been started. The benzodiazepine is able to take the edge off anxiety rapidly, which makes the patient more comfortable and more able to comply with antidepressant treatment and therapy.

GUY

Guy, a forty-two-year-old attorney, came to see us for severe anxiety. He felt that he was emotionally out of control. He had periods of intense nervousness, he had trouble catching his breath, his heart pounded hard against his chest, his hands dripped cold sweat, and his mind was filled with negative, anxious thoughts. Guy could turn any event into a disaster in his mind and was always able to ratchet up his anxiety level a few notches higher. A simple bruise on his child was reason for Guy to start planning for his son's eventual chemotherapy. Routine bills in the mail were prophecies in his mind that bankruptcy was inevitable. His wife was surely making plans to leave him when he saw her speaking to fathers at PTA meetings at the school. Living with the burden of this much anxiety was taking its toll on Guy's health. He was struggling with many physical stress symptoms, including headaches, stomachaches, and back pain. Guy's SPECT study showed marked overactivity in the basal ganglia (they were on fire). Guy had tried several antidepressants that didn't help, so we prescribed a benzodiazepine (Klonopin) for him. Like most patients with moderate to severe anxiety, Guy also needed more support than medication alone, and we also recommended biofeedback and cognitive behavioral therapy (CBT). Within two months of starting treatment he felt much better. He was calmer, less tense, and more in control of his emotions. Over time, with the help of psychotherapy, he was able to slowly taper and stop the Klonopin.

SHERRIE

Sherrie, a thirty-two-year-old business executive, came to see us about her fear of driving. She had not driven a car in ten years. Her husband spent an extra hour and a half each day driving her to and from work in rush-hour traffic. Every time Sherrie got behind the wheel of a car she experienced panic symptoms—heart palpitations; cold, sweaty hands; trouble catching her breath; and muscle tension in her neck. Her thoughts focused on horrific events related to driving, such as being in a fiery accident or running over a child or an animal. In talking to Sherrie we discovered her grandmother also had severe problems with anxiety and did not leave her own home for forty years. Her family physician had tried her on a couple of medications that didn't help. Sherrie's SPECT study showed marked overactivity in the basal ganglia, especially on the left side. We placed her on

Xanax, a benzodiazepine, in addition to teaching her deep-relaxation techniques. When Sherrie had learned to control her tendency to predict panic attacks and had mastered deep relaxation, we started her on a program of "systematic desensitization." The program gradually increased her exposure to driving in a controlled environment. First we had her imagine driving for longer and longer intervals while feeling very relaxed. Within a week she felt less anxious and in better control of her emotions. Gradually she was able to drive for progressively longer periods of time while still employing the self-relaxation techniques. Over the next four months she was able to drive comfortably by herself. Sherrie continued in therapy but slowly tapered and eventually stopped Xanax. Like many patients, she experienced memory problems when taking Xanax at full dose. While she still keeps a few Xanax tablets with her "just in case," she hasn't taken one in three years. Her follow-up SPECT scan off meds, after therapy was markedly improved.

Sherrie's Before and After Treatment

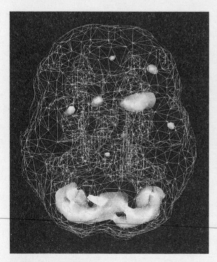 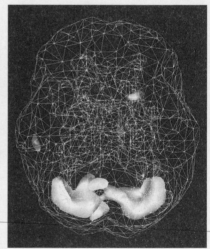

Before treatment
Underside active view
Increased basal ganglia,
especially on left side.

After treatment
Underside active view
Overall calming of basal ganglia
activity.

LES

Les came to the clinic after being on Valium for six years. He said that initially it helped his anxiety attacks, but recently he was experiencing memory and motivational problems. When we scanned him on Valium, the scan showed overall decreased brain activity. Using the information from the scan, we slowly took him off the Valium and replaced it with an antidepressant with anti-anxiety effects. He reported over six months that his memory and motivation improved without an increase in his anxiety.

Les's Scan After Six Years of Valium

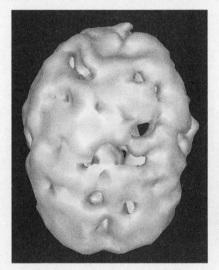

Top-down surface view
Overall decreased activity with
scalloping noted.

Buspirone is a non-benzodiazepine anti-anxiety medication. It may be used alone or prescribed in combination with some of the antidepressants to augment, or increase, their effectiveness. Buspirone must be taken three times daily and needs time to start working. Patients who start on buspirone should understand that the dosage may need to be increased over time in order to derive maximum clinical benefit and that they should expect buspirone to take seven to ten days to start working.

The tricyclic antidepressants imipramine and desipramine are often helpful in treating anxiety disorders, especially panic disorder. Some patients experience "jitteriness" or feel "revved up" the first few days they take an antidepressant. For those with anxiety disorders, feeling more "revved up" can be extremely uncomfortable. To minimize this side effect, we tell our patients what they might experience and we start the medication at the lowest possible dose. The dose is gradually increased as needed and as the patient adjusts to the medication. An anticonvulsant, a benzodiazepine or Buspirone taken along with the antidepressant, may be very helpful if anxiety is severe or incapacitating. Like buspirone, the antidepressants take time to work. During the two- to four-week waiting period, other therapies such as biofeedback and self-relaxation techniques can be extremely helpful in decreasing patient discomfort.

SUSAN

Susan was a twenty-eight-year-old elementary schoolteacher who suffered from chronic anxiety. She felt tense, nervous, restless, and on edge. Susan was often irritable with her family and students and felt overwhelmed by the guilt from her negative behavior. She also had an extreme fear of flying. Her family lived in Minnesota and she felt terrible that she could not travel to Minnesota from California for family gatherings. She had tried the benzodiazepines Valium, Xanax, and Klonopin, but they made her feel dopey. We prescribed the tricyclic antidepressant imipramine at moderate doses. Within two weeks she noticed she felt calmer and more in control of her emotions. She felt as though her emotions matched the situation she was in, rather than having the feeling of being driven by anxiety. In addition to her medication, she was taught biofeedback and deep-relaxation therapy.

Anticonvulsant or antiseizure medications work by stabilizing and calming brain function and often decrease the activity level of the basal ganglia. Anticonvulsants are covered in more detail later in this chapter under the cyclic and temporal lobe types. In our experience, they also tend to work for Type 1, Pure Anxiety. Jack Dreyfus, founder of the famous Dreyfus mutual fund, wrote a book many years ago titled *A Remarkable Medicine Has Been Overlooked* about the effects of the anticonvulsant Dilantin in psychiatry. He had experienced both anxiety and depression and the common medications for those disorders were of no use to him; in fact, they caused bad side effects. When he took the older anticonvulsant Dilantin he quickly noticed that he felt calmer, more relaxed, and significantly better overall. For the past twenty years psychiatrists have been using this class of medication in psychiatry in ever-increasing numbers. The SPECT scans help us understand why. If these disorders were due to areas of nerve cell firing instability, which are like seizures, it would make sense that using anticonvulsants to stabilize nerve cell firing would have beneficial effects for people with anxiety and/or depressive disorders.

NICHOLAS

Nicholas had been plagued with anxiety ever since his days in Vietnam. He felt as though his brain was reset during the war. He felt revved up, tense all over, and on edge. Noises bothered him, he had terrible headaches, and his blood pressure was often elevated. He felt as though he was always waiting for bad things to happen. His wife left him because she had trouble dealing with someone who was "so tightly wound." During a particularly bad week he started thinking about suicide, which was the reason he came to the clinic. His SPECT study showed dramatic hyperactivity in his left basal ganglia, and due to the focal nature of the finding (seen on one side and not the other) he was placed on the anticonvulsant Depakote. In three days he had a dramatically positive response. His headaches improved, he felt significantly less tense, and his level of irritability went from 10 (on a scale from 1 to 10) down to 2. He was also easier to be around. Before his treatment, people avoided Nicholas; he was too on edge for people to be able to enjoy his company. After the Depakote, he was more relaxed and better able to show his compassionate, funny personality.

Type 2: Pure Depression—Hot Deep Limbic System (DLS)

Type 2, Pure Depression is best treated with antidepressant medication that enhances the neurotransmitters norepinephrine and dopamine, such as the tricyclic antidepressants desipramine, imipramine, and buproprion.

Tricyclic antidepressants (TCAs) need to be monitored very carefully because of their effect on heart function. This is extremely important for the elderly, for children, and for people taking multiple medications. Desipramine

Anti-anxiety Meds				
Generic name	Brand name	Milligrams a day/ Available strengths	Times a day	Notes
alprazolam	Xanax	0.25 to 5+/ 0.25, 0.5, 1, 2	1 to 5	Best used for situational panic attacks (fear of flying) and unresponsive anxiety; can be highly addictive. Interacts negatively with some other drugs, like Serzone.
clonazepam	Klonopin	0.5 to 4/ 0.5, 1, 2	2	Long-acting, can be taken twice daily. Anticonvulsant and anti-anxiety properties.
diazepam	Valium	2 to 40/ 2, 5, 10	2 to 4	Intermediate-acting. Muscle relaxant; anticonvulsant and anti-anxiety properties.
buspirone (non-benzo-diazepine)	BuSpar	15 to 60/ 5, 7.5, 15	3	Takes 7 to 10 days to start working. Usually better as an add-on drug rather than a primary treatment in our experience. Nonaddictive.
clorazepate benzodiaze-pine	Tranxene	11.25 to 22.5SD/ 15 to 30 T-Tab/ 11.25, 22.5 SD 3.25, 7.5, 15 T-Tab	1-SD 3-T-Tab	Long-acting, may accumulate and cause sedation. Can be used to help with management of alcohol withdrawal.
lorazepam	Ativan	2 to 6/ 0.5, 1, 2, and injection	1 to 4	Intermediate length of action.

*The tricyclic antidepressants are discussed under Type 2. The anticonvulsants are discussed under Type 6.

has been associated with an increased incidence of sudden cardiac death in children. Therefore, if desipramine is given to pediatric patients, they should have a baseline electrocardiogram (ECG), frequent monitoring, and additional ECGs during follow-up visits. The toxic effect that TCAs exert on the heart explains their danger. These medications are very dangerous in overdose and should never be kept where children or a confused adult may gain access to them. TCAs should not be taken in combination with the pain medication Ultram because of the potential for causing seizures.

Additionally, TCAs may have annoying side effects. They may cause weight gain, sedation, and daytime lethargy. People who take them sometimes complain of gastrointestinal problems such as nausea and constipation. They can also cause dry mouth, blurred vision, shakiness or tremors, dizziness, and sexual dysfunction.

Starting a TCA at the lowest possible dose and then increasing it slowly can minimize side effects. The good news about TCA side effects is that many of them go away on their own within the first few days to weeks of treatment, and the others are usually easily managed. Taking the medication at dinnertime allows it to wear off sooner and decreases daytime drowsiness. Taking the medication with food, increasing fiber in the diet, and increasing fluid intake can help gastrointestinal complaints. Caffeinated beverages such as tea, coffee, and soft drinks do not count as increased fluid intake. Chewing sugar-free gum helps the problem of dry mouth and using eyedrops improves the discomfort of dry eyes. A high-protein, low-carbohydrate diet and a fitness program can help manage weight and improve depression and anxiety.

Like all antidepressants, TCAs take time to start working, and it may be two to four weeks before the symptoms of anxiety and depression begin to abate. Although sleep disturbance, energy levels, and appetite may respond earlier, mood, self-esteem, and one's general outlook may take longer to resolve. In the case of anxiety the full benefit of medication may not be experienced for eight to twelve weeks.

JON

Jon was a fifty-five-year-old engineer referred by his internist for consultation after a medical workup failed to uncover any reason for his insomnia, loss of appetite, weight loss, fatigue, and vague aches and pains. At the clinic, Jon's wife revealed that he had been withdrawn and distant for weeks. Although he appeared to be in emotional pain, his friends and family were unable to engage him in any activities or conversation. He had no interest in previous activities and could barely force himself to go to work. Jon described his mind as "just blank" because it was "work even to think." Once in the past he had briefly felt the same way but had not sought treatment at the time.

Jon's symptoms were those of Pure Depression, and, like many men who suffer with depression, he had not gotten help in the past but instead had "pulled himself up by the bootstraps." Jon's SPECT studies showed markedly increased activity in his limbic system on both his baseline and concentration scans. He couldn't cope with this bout of depression on his own, and he needed the Tofranil (TCA) that we prescribed for him. Within a month both he and his family noticed that he felt more energetic, focused, and was happier and willing to join in with family and friends.

Wellbutrin is unrelated to the TCA and SSRI classes of antidepressants. It is a well-tolerated medication with a strong safety profile. We prescribe Wellbutrin frequently in our clinics because it is a very effective antidepressant and seems to stimulate the prefrontal cortex. In many cases we use it to treat patients with mild cases of ADD, especially when it is mixed with this type of depression. We also use it as an add-on drug to boost the effect of other antidepressants, especially the SSRIs.

Wellbutrin comes in an immediate-release form that should be taken on a twice-daily to three-times-a-day dosing schedule and a sustained-release form that should be taken twice daily. A single dose of the immediate-release form should not exceed 150mg, and a single dose of the sustained-release form should not exceed 150mg. The total daily dose of any form of Wellbutrin should not exceed 450mg.

A side effect of Wellbutrin that most people tend to enjoy is weight loss. It is an energizing medication with positive metabolic effects. Wellbutrin usually does not cause the annoying TCA side effects. People also enjoy the prosexual effects of Wellbutrin. We use it to manage the sexual dysfunction that is caused by other medications.

Wellbutrin has also been extensively studied to assess its potential to lower seizure thresholds in patients. After Wellbutrin was first released, it was taken off the market for further study because of concerns about the increased incidence of seizures in patients taking it. Wellbutrin was determined to be safe after additional studies, but because of the initial concerns, the dosing guidelines should be followed.

CONNIE

After the death of her parents in an automobile accident, thirty-three-year-old Connie had episodes of breaking down into tears, feeling sad for days on end, and she lost interest in life. After nearly a year she despaired that she would ever feel better, and realized she had depression, not simply a grief reaction, and got help. Connie's family doctor gave her 75mg of imipramine (a TCA) to help the symptoms of depression. When she came to see us she did not feel better and complained of dry mouth and constipation. Her SPECT study showed marked increased deep limbic activity. We switched her over to Wellbutrin, due to its superior side-effect profile. In three weeks she noticed she had more energy and had a more positive outlook and an increased desire to see and interact with her family and friends. Her follow-up scan showed significant improvement.

Connie's Before and After Treatment With Wellbutrin

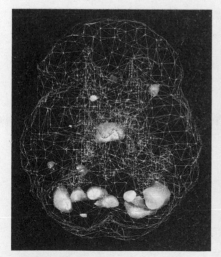 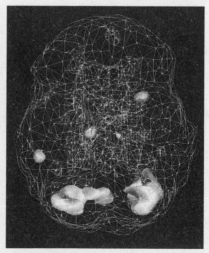

Before treatment
Underside active view
Increased deep limbic system activity.

After treatment
Underside active view
Overall calming of deep limbic system.

Antidepressants for Type 2				
Generic name	Brand name	Milligrams a day/ Available strengths	Times a day	Notes
buproprion	Wellbutrin	50 to 450/ 75, 100	2 to 3	Never give more than 150mg per dose. Do not exceed 450mg per day. Do not use in combination with other drugs that lower seizure threshold if the person is prone to seizures. Excellent for complaints of sexual dysfunction.
buproprion sustained release	Wellbutrin SR	150 to 450/ 100, 150	1 to 2	Never give more than 300mg a dose. Do not exceed 450mg per day. Do not use in combination with other drugs that lower seizure threshold if the person is prone to seizures. Excellent for complaints of sexual dysfunction. The SR tablets should never be divided.
desipramine TCA	Norpramin	100 to 300/ 10, 25, 50, 75, 100, 150	1 to 2	Often very effective but should be used with caution in children because of the risk of sudden cardiac death.
imipramine TCA	Tofranil	10 to 300/ 5, 10, 50, 75, 100, 125, 150	1 to 2	Also used for anxiety, panic disorder, bed-wetting.

Generic name	Brand name	Milligrams a day/ Available strengths	Times a day	Notes
amitriptyline TCA	Elavil	10 to 300/ 10, 25, 50, 75, 100, 150	1 to 2	Very low doses are often used to help with sleep problems, fibromyalgia, and pain syndromes. Higher doses tend to have many side effects.
nortriptyline TCA	Pamelor	10 to 150/ 10, 25, 50, 75	1 to 2	Generally better tolerated than other TCAs. May have a "therapeutic window," which means it may work in a certain dose range but not if you go above or below the effectve dose.
doxepin TCA	Sinequan	10 to 300/ 10, 25, 50, 75, 100, 150	1 to 2	Often used to help with sleep problems.
trimipramine TCA	Surmontil	75 to 200/ 25, 50, 100	1 to 2	Should be given in divided doses.
protriptyline TCA	Vivactil	15 to 60/ 10	1 to 2	Should be given in three to four divided doses. Another of the better-tolerated TCAs. Less sedating than many others.

Type 3: Mixed Anxiety and Depression—Hot BG and DLS

Type 3, Mixed Anxiety and Depression often responds to tricyclic antide-pressants alone or in combination with an anticonvulsant or low dose ben-zodiazepine. Serzone is another choice for this type, but it has recently been given a "black box" warning by the FDA because it has caused liver failure in a small number of cases.

The tricyclic antidepressant imipramine increases both serotonin and norepinephrine. We have found it very helpful when anxiety and depression coexist. Imipramine can be used in combination with buspirone to help treat chronic pain disorders. Patients with chronic pain are at increased risk for developing depression. Many of them have PTSD because their pain is related to an accident or other trauma. Anxiety and depression complicated by increased muscle tension in turn increases pain. A depressed patient cannot fully participate in therapies, medical treatment, and pain management programs. Treatment of depression and anxiety is an extremely important part of any pain management protocol. There is no evidence that antidepressant medications exert effects that decrease pain independent of their antidepressant effects.

MARGARET

Margaret, forty-nine, suffered from fibromyalgia and CFS. She also had a history of several bad relationships with men who had been abusive. Margaret had a history of abuse in childhood, had been depressed off and on for many years and had high levels of anxiety. She hurt all over, emotionally and physically. After many antidepressants, painkillers, and therapists, nothing Margaret tried seemed to help relieve her suffering. Margaret's SPECT scans helped her understand the brain-based reasons for many of her symptoms. Her anxiety centers and her limbic system were extremely overactive, and this increased activity was the driving force behind the anxiety and depression Margaret continued to experience.

Imipramine was a good choice of antidepressant for Margaret because we have had good results in our patient population who suffer from mixed anxiety and depression and because this is one of the antidepressants that sometimes benefits people with chronic pain disorders. Imipramine can often rapidly improve sleep disturbance for patients. This is a very important consideration for patients who are suffering from fibromyalgia, CFS, chronic insomnia, or any medical condition with associated sleep disturbance.

After she was stabilized on imipramine, BuSpar (buspirone) was added to further boost the effect of imipramine and to provide more anxiety reduction. Margaret's emotional and physical discomfort was markedly reduced. She was able to actively participate in physical therapy and a support group.

No discussion about treatment options for anxiety and depression is complete unless a review of the monoamine oxidase inhibitors (MAOIs) is included. The MAOIs are extremely powerful drugs that interfere with the action of an enzyme called monoamine oxidase. Monoamine oxidase breaks down neurotransmitters such as norepinephrine, dopamine, and serotonin. By preventing this enzyme from doing its job, MAOIs may exert their antidepressant effects by allowing neurotransmitters to increase to very high levels in the brain.

Over time, the MAOIs have proved superior to other medications for the treatment of depression complicated by anxiety and other forms of atypical depression. Atypical depressions are characterized by changes in biorhythms that are the opposite of what is usually expected in major depression. People suffering from an atypical depression are likely to have excessive weight gain and an increased appetite rather than no appetite and weight loss. They oversleep and have trouble getting to sleep at night rather than suffering from early morning awakenings. They have more agitation and panic. Another group of depressed patients that tend to respond well to MAOIs are those with rejection sensitivity, very poor self-esteem, and such low energy levels that they feel like they can't move. Patients who are unresponsive to TCAs and the other classes of antidepressants may also benefit from treatment with an MAOI.

MAOIs are not usually the first medication many doctors choose for a patient, even for a patient with an atypical depression. This is because the newer generation of drugs (Prozac, Wellbutrin, and so on) is much easier for doctors to manage, and therefore the medications with history have unfortunately become largely drugs of last resort. Like the TCAs, SSRIs, or any other drug, the MAOIs have their own set of side effects and management problems.

Patients taking MAOIs can minimize side effects by starting the medication and then slowly increasing the dose. MAOIs should be taken in two to three divided doses during the day. One of the most common side effects is postural hypotension. This is low blood pressure that causes a person to feel dizzy when standing up after sitting or lying down for a while and many medications can cause it. Increasing fluids and getting up more slowly usually take care of the problem, but sometimes other interventions are needed. In general, complaints of dry mouth, constipation, lethargy, and blurred vision are less common with MAOIs than with TCAs.

The reason your doctor needs to know her stuff when she recommends an MAOI is not because of their relatively low overall side-effect profile, nor is it because of their proven ability to help a lot of depressions that don't respond to other treatments; it's the need to restrict any substances that release tyramine, epinephrine, dopamine, or norepinephrine. If these substances are increased in your system while you are taking an MAOI, a hypertensive crisis can be produced. Blood pressure rapidly rises to potentially fatal or stroke levels and is often accompanied by severe headache, sweating, nausea, and irregular heartbeats. Emergency treatment is necessary. To avoid a hypertensive crisis, you need to keep high-tyramine-content foods out of your diet, and these include: aged cheeses such as cheddar, Swiss, blue, and Camembert; smoked or pickled meats such as sausage, herring, or corned beef; aged meats, fish, or poultry like pâtés, liver, and game; yeast, meat extracts, brewer's yeast, and stews made with these; red wine, Chianti, burgundy, sherry, and vermouth; Italian broad beans such as fava beans; beers; caffeine including chocolate; soy sauce; yogurt and sour cream; and figs, raisins, grapes, pineapple, and oranges. There are many medications that must be strictly avoided as well because they will also interact with the MAOIs to cause a hypertensive crisis. The most dangerous drugs to avoid are stimulants and cocaine; decongestants; some blood pressure medications; other antidepressants; narcotics; and, if you require anesthesia, your doctors absolutely must know that you are taking an MAOI. Your doctor must be able to educate you fully about the diet plan for MAOIs and you need to be committed to a healthy eating pattern (no cheating). You also have to be willing and able to take the medication three times daily to get the best response. If you can't commit fully to the program, choose another one. Even the best one won't help if you don't work it.

Type 4: Overfocused Anxiety/Depression—Hot Anterior Cingulate Gyrus (ACG) and BG and/or DLS

Type 4, Overfocused Anxiety/Depression is most likely caused by a serotonin deficiency. Medication interventions need to be aimed at this neurotransmitter system. SSRIs focus on enhancing serotonin availability in the brain and calm the anterior cingulate gyrus and basal ganglia.

The release of Prozac in the 1980s revolutionized the treatment of anxiety and depression. Suddenly, physicians had a medication available that was extremely effective in alleviating the primary symptoms of these disorders and it was also well tolerated and easy to prescribe. Patients tolerated Prozac much better than the older tricyclic antidepressant medications and the monoamine

Antidepressants for Type 3				
Generic name	Brand name	Milligrams a day/ Available strengths	Times a day	Notes
nefazodone	Serzone	300 to 600/ 50, 100, 150, 200, 250	1 to 2	Caution must be used due to the recent "black box" warning from the FDA for rare cases of liver failure. Not for use with Tegretol, Orap, Halcion, Propulsid, and Xanax. May cause less sexual dysfunction than SSRIs; used for chronic pain disorders in combination with buspirone.
*desipramine TCA	Norpramin	10 to 300/ 10, 25, 50, 75, 100, 150	1 to 2	Often very effective but should be used with caution in children because of the risk of sudden cardiac death.
*imipramine TCA	Tofranil	10 to 300/ 10, 25, 50, 75, 100, 125, 150	1 to 2	Also used for anxiety, panic disorder, bed-wetting.
phenelzine monoamine oxidase inhibitor MAOI	Nardil	45 to 90/ 15	3	Most commonly used MAOI. Very serious drug-drug interactions with many compounds including the SSRIs and some pain medications; requires diet restriction because of interaction with tyramine in foods.
tranylcypromine MAOI	Parnate	30 to 60/ 10	3	Same restrictions as above.

*These medications are also discussed in the section covering Type 2.

inhibitors because it caused very few side effects and did not have dietary interactions. Physicians liked it because it was a very safe medication. They could prescribe it without worrying so much about the blood pressure and cardiac effects of the older medications, the potential disastrous consequences of overdose, or hassling with complicated dosing and titration schedules. There are now several SSRI medications besides Prozac available for use.

The use of antidepressants, especially the SSRIs, is increasing. This is because we are now using them to treat many disorders besides depression. Antidepressants are used to treat anxiety disorders, headache conditions, some forms of ADHD, premenstrual syndromes, and chronic pain disorders, to name just a few. The overall improved tolerability of the newer generation antidepressants has contributed to the increasing use of antidepressants. Many other factors have amplified the number of antidepressant prescriptions that are written annually, including increased patient request for treatment driven by direct-to-consumer marketing and education efforts of pharmaceutical companies, greater focus by primary care physicians on mental health issues, and the lessening of the stigma previously associated with psychoactive drug use.

The more the drugs are used, the more we have learned about them. We know with absolute certainty that there is still no "magic bullet" available. All drugs, even aspirin, have side effects. Medications have side effects because, unlike heat-seeking missiles that are true to their intended targets, they, and their metabolites, scatter. They scatter throughout the brain and the body, attaching to receptors indiscriminately, to both those they should influence and those they should not. This scatter effect and unwanted influence on targets other than the primary targets are what result in the unwanted side effects of medications.

The SSRI antidepressants have far fewer side effects in general than most other antidepressants. They do not cause significant delay of electrical impulses through the heart and therefore are much safer in cases of accidental or intentional overdose. This is very important when we are considering prescribing an antidepressant for a suicidal patient. It is just as important when we are treating a medically compromised patient, an elderly patient who may get confused and accidentally take an extra dose, or when there are children at home who may gain access to drugs. Blood pressure is usually not significantly affected by SSRIs and this is again an important consideration for older patients, those taking several medications, and for anyone prone to dizziness.

Most SSRIs can be taken in a single daily dose. Once-a-day dosing boosts compliance with treatment. People have trouble remembering to take medications multiple times each day. The more complicated a medication dosing schedule is, the more likely treatment is to fail. People also do not like to be reminded of illness. They would rather be able to take a medication as infrequently as possible. An exception to the single daily dosing schedule for SSRIs is Luvox, which should be given twice a day when the total daily dose exceeds 100mg.

SSRIs avoid most of the common and uncomfortable side effects that the older medications caused, such as blurred vision, gastrointestinal disturbances, weight gain, sedation, dry mouth, constipation, and palpitations (skipped heartbeats). In clinical practice, Luvox can cause stomach upset at higher doses, and Paxil tends to generate more complaints of weight gain and sedation than the other SSRIs.

SSRI medications sometimes cause people to feel jittery or nervous for the first few days after the medication is started. This is a normal response to the medication and usually resolves within one to two weeks. If it is very uncomfortable, the dose may be lowered slightly for a few days to allow the medication level to rise more slowly.

There is a large body of literature supporting the safety profile of Prozac use during pregnancy and lactation. Children born to women who took Prozac during their pregnancy are at no greater risk of any negative birth event or developmental problem than children born to women in the general population. And women who take Prozac are at no greater risk of pregnancy complications than women in the general population. We do know children born to women with untreated psychiatric conditions have a much higher incidence of learning disorders, behavioral disorders, and attachment issues. The other SSRI medications are probably safe, but there is not yet as much data and literature in support of their use in pregnancy and breast-feeding.

Sexual dysfunction is a common complaint among patients taking antidepressant medication. But when exactly can we know this is a side effect of medications? We have learned through our work with patients how difficult this question can be to answer.

Sexual dysfunction is an issue our patients rarely bring up early in the therapeutic relationship and almost never mention during the first visit. They are overwhelmed with anxiety or the symptoms of depression and feel compelled to tell us about those concerns. They are almost always focused on getting relief from anxiety, insomnia, fatigue, and sadness as the primary goals of the visit. We are busy with the work of making sure our patients are not suicidal, do not have a major neurological or medical illness, and are not struggling with the complication of substance abuse. We are reviewing the results of their evaluation, brain SPECT imaging procedures, and developing a treatment plan.

Sexual dysfunction is initially low on everyone's priority list. This changes as the initial target symptoms start to improve. Our patients return to us and report the problem of sexual dysfunction. We must determine whether this is a lingering symptom of the underlying condition or, indeed, a side effect of treatment. We have learned that a well-documented history of sexual functioning obtained prior to the initiation of medication management helps us make this distinction.

The most common sexual complaints patients on antidepressants have are failure of arousal and orgasm dysfunction. Since all antidepressants, with the exception of Wellbutrin, reportedly cause sexual dysfunction to some degree, management of this side effect is critical. There are several strategies to consider.

When an antidepressant is working well (target symptoms are responding) but sexual dysfunction becomes an issue, we may initially counsel our patient to wait for spontaneous resolution of the side effect. Most medication side effects go away on their own within the first twelve weeks of treatment, and this happens occasionally with the complaint of sexual dysfunction.

When waiting for a reasonable period of time doesn't cause the side effect to resolve, we frequently use adjunctive, or secondary, compounds to help reduce the problem. Some people derive great benefit from these agents and others do not. Management of this side effect is an art and must be individualized.

Wellbutrin has prosexual effects. It may be added to antidepressant treatment protocols to enhance sexual functioning and boost performance of the other antidepressant. For example, a woman taking Sarafem (fluoxetine) for PMS and anxiety may be very pleased with the overall effectiveness of Sarafem in alleviating her initial symptoms. She may also be experiencing sexual dysfunction as a common SSRI side effect. The addition of Wellbutrin 100mg SR–150mg SR daily is likely to eliminate the sexual dysfunction complaint. Wellbutrin is very well tolerated, has a very low side-effect profile, has very few drug-drug interactions, and is our favorite agent for the treatment of sexual dysfunction.

Buspirone (BuSpar) is a non-benzodiazepine anxiolytic medication that is commonly used to treat anxiety. It is also used in combination with antidepressants to augment, or boost, their effectiveness. The reviews concerning the effectiveness of buspirone in alleviating sexual dysfunction have been mixed. If anxiety is the causal factor, or is still contributing significantly, to problems with sexual performance, buspirone might be worth trying. Patients need to know that this is a medication that must be given on a divided dosage schedule, usually three times daily, and the dose almost always needs to be increased a few times for best response. There is also a seven- to ten-day waiting period for buspirone to build a blood level and start working.

Ginkgo biloba is a widely used secondary agent for the treatment of sexual dysfunction, however most of the studies of ginkgo biloba are not well designed. They lack placebo control and other standard methods of selection of subjects and review of results.

Sildenafil (Viagra) remains popular as a treatment for sexual dysfunction caused by medications. A recent study by Salerian, et al, included both men and women in a study of the use of Viagra for medication-induced sexual dysfunction. In this study, patients had sexual dysfunction related to various psychoactive medications (mood stabilizers, TCAs, atypical antipsychotics, SSRIs, benzodiazepines, and so on) and most of them were taking two or more of these medications. Each patient took Viagra (average dose—50mg) for one to thirty-six weeks. Eighty-eight percent of the men and women reported overall improvement regardless of the type of psychoactive medication they were taking. The patients who were taking SSRI drugs reported slightly less improvement than the other patients. There have been several other small studies of the effect of Viagra on medication-induced sexual dysfunction in women that have been mostly positive.

Viagra should be used with great caution when patients have heart problems, blood pressure problems, or are taking medications that increase the blood level of Viagra. There is also some evidence that some ethnic groups compared to white males metabolize Viagra differently. There have also been rare reports in the literature of Viagra inducing delusions and other psychiatric complications in elderly males.

We do not recommend "drug holidays" to treat medication-induced sexual dysfunction. We spend the majority of our time teaching patients the importance of adhering to a very strict dosage schedule because we know that medications must be available to the brain in order to be helpful. The timing of some medication schedules is more critical than others. For instance, you might be able to skip a couple of doses of Prozac and not suffer much in the way of consequences because of its very long half-life. Prozac's metabolites live in your system for a long time, exerting their antidepressant and anti-anxiety effects and preventing withdrawal symptoms. However, if you skip a dose of Paxil or Effexor, you are at risk of experiencing withdrawal side effects. We also worry about patients remembering to restart their medication if they skip some doses. In that case, our patient would face the reemergence of their anxiety and depression, potentially derailing weeks or months of hard work and recovery. Finally, we have seen no evidence of the effectiveness of "drug holidays." Having patients skip their morning dose of an antidepressant hasn't produced fireworks later in the evening.

Dose reduction is another approach to treating sexual dysfunction caused by medications. The antidepressant dose can be decreased to see if that causes the side effect to resolve. However, we don't often recommend this approach either because we frequently see a patient seesawing between a dose that treats the illness but causes side effects and a dose that causes fewer side effects but allows symptoms to break through. It is usually better to change antidepressants or add a medication to treat the sexual dysfunction.

THOMAS

Thomas was a twenty-three-year-old college student with a history of temper tantrums in childhood. His grade performance had always been good, but he had trouble relaxing. He described himself as being "high-strung" and a perfectionist by nature. When Thomas got a thought in his mind, he had trouble letting go of it. Struggling with homesickness while away at college, he found himself dwelling on sad thoughts. His mood was depressed and anxious, his energy level was down, and he was spending lots of time chasing the same thought around and around in his mind. Thomas's self-confidence was eroding, and his outlook on life was becoming increasingly negative. His SPECT studies showed overactivity of the limbic system, basal ganglia, and anterior cingulate gyrus on his baseline scan. On his concentration scan, Thomas's anterior cingulate gyrus had even more activity. The more he concentrated, the worse this area of his brain performed.

Because Thomas had overfocused anxiety and depression, we treated him with Prozac because the SSRI medications treat both the overfocused symptoms and depression. Thomas liked the idea of being able to take a medicine only once a day, and he had an excellent emotional response to Prozac. However, over time he complained of concentration and motivation problems. A follow-up scan showed that, while the medication had calmed his emotional brain, it had also calmed his prefrontal cortex, giving him issues with memory and motivation. The follow-up scan helped us realize we needed to lower his dose of Prozac.

Thomas's Before and After Treatment with Prozac

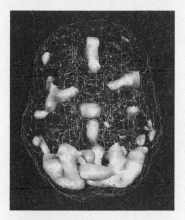 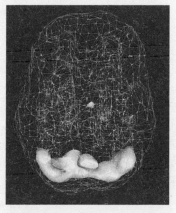

Before treatment
Underside active view
Increased anterior cingulate gyrus,
BG, and DLS.

After treatment
Underside active view
Overall calming of the anterior
cingulate gyrus, BG, and DLS.

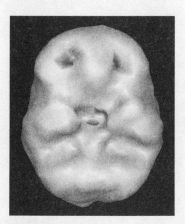 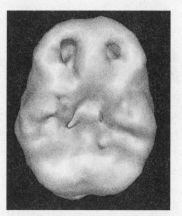

Before treatment
Underside surface view
Overall full surface activity.

After treatment
Underside surface view
Note decreased prefrontal cortex activity.

Ann

Ann came to the clinic for an evaluation because she just "couldn't let go."
This thirty-nine-year-old mother of two had been able to balance the demands of her middle-management position in the computer industry with

those of her family until she started having panic attacks. Ann had always been extremely well organized, and, in fact, if things were out of place it drove her nuts. She described herself as a brooding person who tended to be a "worrywart." During the few months before she came to see us, Ann had been experiencing gradually increasing levels of tension and anxiety. Finally she started to panic, and thoughts that she might have another panic attack got stuck in her mind. She "couldn't let go."

Ann's SPECT studies showed markedly increased activity in her basal ganglia on baseline and concentration and increased activity in her anterior cingulate gyrus on baseline that further increased with concentration.

We started Ann on an SSRI to decrease the activity in her anterior cingulate gyrus and to treat her panic attacks. To minimize the chance that Ann, like many anxiety disorder patients, would experience a brief rise in agitation or anxiety when the SSRI was first started, we started at a very low dose and increased it slowly. After two months Ann was no longer worrying about having panic attacks and was pleasantly surprised when people told her she was easier to be around and to work with.

ALICIA

Alicia recognized the symptoms of anxiety and depression because her twin sister had been treated for them in the past. Like her sister, Alicia also tended to be stubborn. She liked to have things go her way and found herself frequently picking fights with her family and friends over fairly insignificant events. Whenever she got angry it took her a long time to calm down, and if she was later reminded of the anger-provoking episode she would think about it again for days. Alicia's SPECT scan showed increased limbic system activity and increased anterior cingulate gyrus activity.

Alicia needed an antidepressant to calm her limbic and anterior gyrus activity levels. Alicia started on Zoloft, which made a remarkable difference for her. She was less tense and no longer felt at the mercy of her anger; she could calm down more easily and stopped picking fights. Her thinking was more flexible, and she saw more options in situations and had a more positive outlook. Her mood lifted and the depressive symptoms resolved.

These cases illustrate the additional positive impact that the SSRI medications may have. In addition to treating the symptoms of anxiety and depression, SSRI medications also help improve several areas of personality functioning: They help people have a more positive outlook, decrease irritability, improve energy levels, and decrease some forms of aggression. People become less brooding and inflexible in their thought processes on SSRI medications. Children with temper tantrums, especially when they are the result of people telling them no, may be helped by SSRIs.

Of note, as with other medications, when SSRIs are given to people for the wrong type of anxiety and depression, they can make things much worse. For example, SSRIs tend to make people with Type 5, Cyclic Anxiety/Depression, or Type 6, Temporal Lobe Anxiety/Depression, more emotionally unstable. We have also seen them make these types more irritable and, on occasion, more aggressive. They tend to make people with Type 7, Unfocused Anxiety/Depression, less motivated and less focused.

Another option for overfocused symptoms is Anafranil. Anafranil (clomipramine) is a tricyclic antidepressant that was approved for the treatment of OCD several years before the development of SSRIs. Because it causes the same side effects that the TCAs do, Anafranil is usually reserved for use as a second-line drug (after the SSRIs) for the treatment of OCD and other severe anxiety disorders. It is also commonly used to augment, or boost, the effect of SSRIs for treatment of these same disorders.

Here is a list of the current SSRIs at the time of press.

Selective Serotonin Reuptake Inhibitors (SSRIs)				
Generic name	Brand name	Milligrams a day/ Available strengths	Times a day	Notes
fluoxetine SSRI	Prozac	10 to 80+ 10, 20 (Also available in a once-weekly dosage form [Prozac Weekly], a liquid, and a scored 10mg tablet that can be divided into 5mg)	1	Long-acting, stays in body up to six weeks after last dose. Has been approved for eating disorders, PMS, and OCD. Generally regarded as the safest antidepressant in pregnancy/lactation. Dr. Routh's first choice among the SSRIs.

Generic name	Brand name	Milligrams a day/ Available strengths	Times a day	Notes
fluoxetine SSRI	Sarafem	10 to 20/ 10, 20	1	Approved for treatment of depression and anxiety related to hormonal imbalance, such as PMS.
sertraline SSRI	Zoloft	25 to 200/ 25, 50, 100	1	Usually Dr. Amen's first choice among the SSRIs. Also available in a liquid form. May be associated with a discontinuation syndrome upon suddenly stopping the medication; patients may experience nausea, diarrhea, headache, dizziness, or even disorientation.
paroxetine SSRI	Paxil	10 to 60; lower for elderly and children/ 10, 20, 30, 40	1	Often associated with a discontinuation syndrome, which tends to be more severe in our experience than Zoloft; also available in liquid form.
fluvoxamine SSRI	Luvox	100 to 300 adults; 50 to 200 children/ 25, 50, 100	1	Also approved for OCD.
citalopram SSRI	Celexa	20 to 60 adults; lower for elderly and children/ 10, 20, 40	1	Also available in a liquid form.
escitalopram	Lexapro	10 to 20/ 10, 20	1	Lexapro is a molecule very similar to Celexa.

Type 5: Cyclic Anxiety/Depression—Focal
Hot Spots in the BG and/or DLS

Type 5 is often treated with a combination of medications. It is one of the types for which we need to carefully individualize a medication treatment plan. Patients with cyclic patterns have triggers with varying levels of sensitivity that, when activated, can provoke another phase of their cycle. One of these triggers may be medication. Medications that are energizing or stimulating might trigger a manic phase. Medications that are slow to work might allow break-through hypomania, mania, anxiety, or depression. The wrong medication for the wrong disorder or patient might make the condition worse or cause the patient to drop out of treatment prematurely because of side effects or the belief that medication won't work.

Our primary objective is to treat depression and stop a cyclic pattern when we see one. In our experience, cycling is best controlled with one of the anticonvulsants. If our patient is also depressed, we add an antidepressant. Sometimes, cycling is not so easily controlled and in those cases we use one of the "atypical or new antipsychotic medications." The atypical or new antipsychotic medications, such as Abilify, Clozaril, Geodon, Risperdal, Zyprexa, and Seroquel, are different from the traditional antipsychotic medications in several fundamental ways. They are drugs that more specifically target the receptor sites involved with psychosis and mood instability, and several of them also have action at the serotonin receptor sites and help with mood. These can be used alone or in combination with the anticonvulsants and antidepressants.

The most important thing to remember when using multiple medications is that, whenever possible, only one medication at a time should be started. This is so that you and your doctor will know which medication is the source of any side effects that might occur. The second most important thing to remember when you are using multiple medications is that you absolutely must inform all of your doctors of every medication you are taking, including all herbal supplements and over-the-counter drugs. These compounds can cause interactions with medications.

The anticonvulsants are discussed under Type 6. The antidepressants are discussed under Types 2, 3, and 4.

Lithium is often prescribed for Cyclic Anxiety/Depression. It is a drug that people most readily associate with psychiatry. Lithium has been around for a very long time and has been used to treat many medical, neurological, and psychiatric disorders. It is one of the best-studied psychiatric medicines available.

Blood work is required when prescribing lithium. We do it initially to establish a therapeutic level of lithium and to check baseline thyroid and kidney function status. Lithium dosage can be increased every five days until a therapeutic level is reached and then the dose can be maintained. Thyroid and kidney function (creatinine level) needs to be checked annually because lithium can decrease the ability of both of these organs to work. In the case of thyroid dysfunction, a patient may continue on lithium therapy with thyroid hormone replacement or switch to an anticonvulsant and add thyroid hormone replacement if needed. However, if the kidneys' ability to function begins to deteriorate, the patient needs to be switched to an anticonvulsant.

Lithium can cause the infamous "lithium tremor," which is really frustrating for anyone who develops it. Lithium tremor causes people's hands to shake and wreaks havoc with their handwriting and any other tasks for which

Lithium Preparations				
Generic name	Brand name	Milligrams a day/ Available strengths	Times a day	Notes
lithium carbonate	Eskalith	For all lithium compounds, total dose is established by blood levels 300	3	Needs to be taken three times daily.
lithium carbonate	Eskalith CR	450	2	Long-acting, can be taken twice daily.
lithium carbonate	generic lithium	150, 300, 600	3	Needs to be taken three times daily.
lithium carbonate	Lithobid Slow- Release Tablets	300	2	Twice daily schedule.
lithium citrate	generic lithium	syrup in liquid form	3	Liquid form that can be given to children, the elderly, and others who can't/won't swallow tablets.

they need smooth hand control. It may also cause nausea, diarrhea, and increased thirst. These milder side effects sometimes get better or go away within the first few days. They can be minimized by taking lithium with food, increasing fluid intake, and using one of the long-acting compounds.

Devon was thirteen but looked much younger than his age. He had

Antipsychotics				
Generic name	Brand name	Milligrams a day/ Available strengths	Times a day	Notes
aripiprazole	Abilify	10 to 30 mg/ 10, 15, 20, 30	1	Newest atypical antipsychotic. Once a day dosing.
olanzapine	Zyprexa Zyprexa Zydis (orally disintegrating tablets)	2.5 to 20/ 2.5, 5, 7.5, 10, 15, 20	1	Atypical antipsychotic, also approved for use in Bipolar Disorder. Once-daily dosing. Very low risk of serious side effects (tardive dyskinesia), improves mood and thought processes.
risperidone	Risperdal	1 to 16/ 0.25, 0.5, 1, 2, 3, 4, and liquid form	1 to 2	At low to moderate doses, acts like an atypical antipsychotic with low side-effect profile. At higher doses, acts like a conventional antipsychotic, and incidence of side effects increases. Not very sedating.
ziprasidone	Geodon	40 to 160/ 20, 40, 60, 80	2	Atypical antipsychotic, generally well tolerated, but may cause greater incidence of blood pressure and heart rhythm problems than other drugs in this class.

Generic name	Brand name	Milligrams a day/ Available strengths	Times a day	Notes
haloperidol	Haldol	Maximum dose is based on clinical response/ 0.5, 1, 2, 5, 10, 20, and immediate and long-acting injection forms	2 to 3	A commonly used conventional anti-psychotic. Approved for use in children. Patients should be monitored for side effects, especially tardive dyskinesia. Very potent and helpful for crisis management.
pimozide	Orap	2 to 10/ 1, 2	2	Used most commonly for the treatment of Tourette's syndrome. Should not be used in combination with antifungal medications or protease inhibitors; used to treat HIV.
clozapine	Clozaril	300 to 900/ 25, 100	3	Atypical antipsychotic requiring weekly blood work. Like Zyprexa, very low incidence of tardive dyskinesia.
quetiapine fumarate	Seroquel	50 to 800/ 25, 100, 200, 300	2	Atypical antipsychotic. Rare reports of effect on thyroid function and cataract formation. Usually well tolerated.

mild mental retardation and previously had been good-natured. Since puberty he had become prone to outbursts of aggression. He was easily frustrated and his behavior seemed to be regressing. Teachers were worried that he would injure himself or someone nearby if he didn't get his way. He wasn't learning the way he had been the year before. Additionally, Devon seemed more resistant to bathing and hygiene. He also seemed angry, sad, and sometimes both, and he was impatient and difficult to console.

Devon responded well to lithium. His mood improved and his behavioral outbursts decreased. The escalating nature of his aggression was stopped. Lithium is a very effective medication for the treatment of aggression, cyclic mood pattern, and suicidal thought patterns. Medications that can be used as alternatives or in addition to lithium are the anticonvulsants and antipsychotics.

Conventional antipsychotics such as Thorazine and Haldol have many side effects. The most common physical complaints are dry mouth, gastrointestinal complaints, fatigue, sedation, and muscle aches. Mentally, people complain about feeling like they have no motivation, as though their mind were blank or they were in a dense fog. These medications also cause a restless condition called akathisia in which people feel the need to shuffle their feet and pace. People can sometimes look as though they have parkinsonism because of the tremors, muscle rigidity, and expressionless look they develop. Finally, the conventional antipsychotics are associated with more serious conditions such as tardive dyskinesia.

Tardive dyskinesia is a movement disorder that can be caused by exposure to antipsychotic medications. The movements are involuntary, meaning that people cannot control them, and are potentially irreversible. The risk of tardive dyskinesia may be increased by the length of time a person has been taking an antipsychotic and by the dose. Higher doses for long periods of time may be riskier than a brief course of treatment with a low dose. The risk of tardive dyskinesia is especially great for elderly women.

It is important to realize that most, if not all, of the antipsychotics and related medications can cause tardive dyskinesia and it can happen at any time during treatment. There is no known treatment for tardive dyskinesia. So how do we help our patients manage this potential problem?

Education is very important. Patients and family members need to know that tardive dyskinesia starts with movements of the tongue and mouth. We look for this and examine our patients when they come to the clinic and we have them self-monitor. We use the lowest possible dose of medication for the shortest period of time and only when the condition warrants its use. And, most important, we select a medication that we believe to be one of the safest, based on current evidence.

Clozaril was the first atypical antipsychotic developed and introduced in 1975. Atypical antipsychotics are also called new generation, novel, or unconventional antipsychotics. Clozaril avoids causing many of the negative muscle and movement reactions (also called extrapyramidal side effects) that the conventional antipsychotics cause and it has not been associated with tardive dyskinesia. But it did not turn out to be the wonder drug as hoped for. Unfortunately, Clozaril poses a significant risk of agranulocytosis, a life-threatening drop in neutrophil (white blood cell) count, and therefore patients must have weekly blood work done. It also increases the risk for seizures, drops in blood pressure (orthostatic blood pressure changes), and fainting. We now reserve it for use in patients who need an antipsychotic but who cannot take any of the others.

The pharmaceutical industry continued to refine antipsychotic medications, looking for a drug with the potency of Haldol, the lack of potential to cause tardive dyskinesia and extrapyramidal side effects, and that was also safer than Clozaril. Zyprexa, the result of their efforts, was the next atypical antipsychotic available. Zyprexa has a very low overall side-effect profile, the tardive dyskinesia risk is markedly reduced, and agranulocytosis has not been associated with its use. Blood work does not have to be monitored. As Zyprexa became more popular, other benefits besides decreasing psychotic symptoms became evident. It also acted like a mood stabilizer and mild antidepressant. People who switched to Zyprexa from other antipsychotics rated their quality of life as much improved because they felt more mentally alert, productive at work, and able to socialize.

Many additional atypical antipsychotics have been developed since Zyprexa, including Geodon and Seroquel. These medications are also usually better tolerated than the conventional antipsychotics. People taking Seroquel need to be aware that it has caused cataract development in dogs and lens changes in humans. How Seroquel affects the eye and whether or not Seroquel is actually directly related to these changes is unknown. However, it is recommended that anyone thinking about taking Seroquel have an eye exam, including a slit lamp examination, prior to starting the medication and every six months during treatment. Seroquel may also decrease levels of total and free thyroid hormone (T4). This happens in what we call a dose-dependent manner, meaning it happens more frequently with higher doses of Seroquel. Most of the time, a low T4 stays within the low average range for patients and thyroid-stimulating hormone (TSH) remains normal. Thyroid-stimulating hormone is a better test of whether or not someone is experiencing thyroid dysfunction. However, some patients have had abnormalities of both T4 and TSH and have required hormone replacement.

Geodon is also well tolerated and in general does not cause many side effects. However, it has a tendency to increase the risk of blood pressure changes and heart rhythm abnormalities somewhat more than other medications in this class. Geodon may also be associated with an increased risk of causing a serious rash that necessitates stopping the drug.

Risperdal is another antipsychotic we frequently prescribe at our clinics. Risperdal behaves like the atypical antipsychotics when prescribed in low to moderate doses. In this dosage range, it has few side effects, a low rate of inducing serious complications, and it is not sedating and is well tolerated overall. At higher doses, Risperdal starts to act like the conventional antipsychotics and causes the same sort of problems and side effects you would expect from those older agents.

For our patients who need an antipsychotic medication, we use the newer atypical antipsychotics whenever possible. This reduces the risk of tardive dyskinesia, extrapyramidal side effects, and other movement disorders. We also educate our patients to watch for the onset of any movement disorder and to report any symptoms immediately to their physician. But even the best antipsychotic medications available are not free of side effects and we still need to treat them when they occur. The most common complaint associated with antipsychotic medications, in fact with many medications, is weight gain. The debate rages on as to whether or not medications actually cause weight gain or weight gain is a function of some other underlying condition. We do know that at least half of the adults in the United States are overweight and one in five can be classified as obese. We know that obesity among children and adults in our country is reaching epidemic proportions. So whether or not you are taking a medication, diet and fitness goals should be part of your life plan. Having said that, there are things we can offer our patients to minimize weight gain on antipsychotic medications.

First and foremost, we have all of our patients change their diet and fitness goals. Second, if needed, an H2 blocker (Axid 300mg, not 150mg, or cimetadine) should be added. This addition is especially effective when Zyprexa is prescribed. Patients also need to be screened for unresolved symptoms of depression or binge eating that may be the cause of weight gain. If these are present, an SSRI or Wellbutrin may be effective. Last, if the other interventions are not effective, amantadine 100 to 300mg daily may be helpful. None of these interventions is likely to be effective in the absence of a consistent exercise program and a high-protein diet.

Zoe, nineteen, a sophomore at a local Christian college, was brought to our clinic by her parents. She was not sleeping, had not eaten for several days, and was spending most of her time reading her Bible. Once before Zoe had had a manic episode that started the same way. Zoe was preoccupied with thoughts about good and evil and messages from God, and she saw "patterns" everywhere. She connected words from songs on the radio to phrases in the Bible and deciphered special meanings. Zoe's mood varied from irritable to intensely sad, depending on what the decoded messages meant.

Zoe's SPECT scan showed increased activity of her basal ganglia and mild to moderate patchy uptake across her cortical surface. Zoe could understand that she needed medication management but had misgivings because of her prior experiences with treatment. She had developed a variety of side effects when she was treated with lithium, including a rather severe tremor that interfered with her writing skills. She rejected several medications because of something she had read or for fear of weight gain. We discussed several strategies for managing side effects with Zoe. She chose to take Zyprexa along with an H2 blocker (Axid) to decrease the chance of weight gain.

After four weeks Zoe was feeling like herself again and we talked with her about long-term management of her disorder. She agreed to try some of the newer anticonvulsants and found that she did well on Lamictal. She was then able to taper and stop the Zyprexa. Zoe was also referred for therapy to learn to manage some of her stressors and triggers for mania, hypomania, and depression.

Type 6: Temporal Lobe Anxiety/Depression—Erratic Temporal Lobe Firing and Hot BG and/or DLS

The medications used to treat Type 6, Temporal Lobe Anxiety/Depression are classified as anticonvulsant medications. We do not mean to imply that patients with Temporal Lobe Anxiety/Depression have a seizure disorder. Rather, they have dysfunction in a part of the brain commonly associated with seizures. We have observed the usefulness of these drugs in stabilizing temporal lobe activity and reducing aggression, mood instability, and headaches. In some cases learning problems have improved with anticonvulsant use. Anticonvulsants are often combined with antidepressant medications or other psychoactive medications to achieve an enhanced therapeutic effect. Patients do not need to have a seizure disorder to derive benefit from treatment with an anticonvulsant or antiseizure medication. Often we do not have to prescribe antiseizure dosages for the medication to be effective; sometimes even very small doses are all that is necessary. Anticonvulsants enhance the neurotransmitter GABA, which has a calming or inhibitory effect on nerve cells. In the last twenty years, psychiatry has revolutionized the use of anticonvulsants by extending their application to treat Bipolar Disorder, aggression, and anxiety and to boost the effect of other medications. Psychiatrists now prescribe anticonvulsants almost as frequently as do neurologists.

Anticonvulsants are great medications with many uses and benefits. We tend to favor the newer compounds because they are much easier to manage. Neurontin, Lamictal, Gabatril, Trileptal, and Topamax do not require blood level monitoring and their side-effect profile is superior to that of the older compounds.

Anticonvulsants				
Generic name	Brand name	Milligrams a day/ Available strengths	Times a day	Notes
carbamaze-pine	Carbatrol (slow release only); Tegretol (regular and slow release)	100 to 1,200/ Carbatrol 200, 300 Tegretol 200 Tegretol 100 chew-tab Tegretol XR 100, 200, 400 Tegretol suspension	2 to 3	Very effective in our experience, but it is essential to monitor white blood cell counts and blood levels.
valproic acid	Depakene	125 to 3,000/ 250	1 to 2	Very effective, but need to monitor liver function and blood levels.
divalproate	Depakote (regular and extended release)	125 to 3,000/ 125, 250, 500, 500 extended release	1 to 2	Very effective, but need to monitor liver function and blood levels.
gabapentin	Neurontin	100 to 6,000/ 100, 300, 400, 600, 800, and suspension	1 to 2	Becoming more popular. Nontoxic but wide dosage range.

Generic name	Brand name	Milligrams a day/ Available strengths	Times a day	Notes
topiramate	Topamax	50 to 400/ 15, 25, 100, 200	1 to 2	Has been shown to help decrease weight. In doses over 300mg may cause memory problems. May also cause cataracts and increase the risk of kidney stone formation.
lamotrigine	Lamictal	25 to 500/ 25, 100, 150, 200	1 to 2	Start at 25mg or less and increase slowly. Has antidepressant effects and causes less confusion and memory loss than others.
tiagabine HCl	Gabatril	4 to 32/ 2, 4, 12, 16, 20	1 to 2	Should be increased slowly (weekly intervals) and needs to be taken two to four times daily.
oxcarbazepine	Trileptal	600 to 1,200 adults; based on body wt for children/ 150, 300, 600, and suspension	1 to 2	Needs to be given twice daily. Dose may be increased by weekly intervals.
phenytoin	Dilantin (regular and extended release)	30 to 300/ 30, 50,100 regular 30, 100, 200, 300 extended form; also available in liquid form	1 to 2	Monitor blood levels. Dental hygiene is important since Dilantin causes problems with gums.

Any medication in this class may cause sedation. Like most side effects, sedation will get better with time. Sedation will increase if the dose of an anticonvulsant is increased rapidly, if more than one anticonvulsant is being used, or if additional sedating medications of any kind are also taken. Patients should also be aware that herbal compounds might be sedating. Alcohol and marijuana use will also compound the problem of sedation. The newer generation of anticonvulsants are generally less sedating than the older ones, and Lamictal may be the least sedating of the group.

Another significant complaint people have about the anticonvulsants is their tendency to cause what we call "cognitive impairment." Cognitive impairment is what people mean when they say they are "in a fog." Concentration, attention span, and memory may be impaired, and in the worst cases people may be confused. Again, this is usually more of a problem with the older drugs, when high doses of the newer drugs are used, and when medications are combined. Topamax is an exception. It can cause rather severe cognitive impairment at even low to moderate doses. Lamictal is an exception, too. It does not seem to cause cognitive impairment.

Tegretol is one of the older anticonvulsants. When treatment is started, blood level monitoring is essential to establish a therapeutic level and to check for any adverse bone marrow effects. Blood checks need to be done periodically during the maintenance phase as well. For patients who have more severe cases of cyclic mood disorders, aggression, or serious temporal lobe dysfunction, this is our favorite medication.

Anticonvulsants should not be stopped suddenly because of the risk of withdrawal seizures. The risk increases for patients who are on high doses of anticonvulsants, who have taken them for a prolonged period of time, or who are on multiple medications. Even patients who do not have a seizure disorder may experience a withdrawal seizure if drug levels drop precipitously.

In addition to anticonvulsants, we often use memory-enhancing medication for people with temporal lobe problems. Memory problems are very common in this type. Donepezil (Aricept) is a medication indicated for Alzheimer's disease that works by increasing the amount of acetylcholine in the brain. Acetylcholine is a neurotransmitter that is known to be involved in laying down new memories. Many of our patients with Type 6 who also complain of memory problems have experienced improved memory performance when taking Aricept in addition to their other prescribed treatment.

Doug was a fifty-one-year-old truck driver who had experienced the onset of depression six months after an accident in which he suffered a closed head injury. Doug hit his head against the driver's-side door window and remembers having a mild concussion. In addition to having trouble going to sleep and staying asleep, loss of appetite, mood disturbance, and disinterest in his usual activities, Doug was also having some atypical symptoms. He had headaches that troubled him often and waves of nausea that weren't always associated with the headaches or with anything he ate. He thought that his vision was different, but he couldn't quite describe the problem. At times he thought his eyesight was dimmer or that he saw shadows. Doug's medical doctor had not found anything unusual during Doug's last several visits. Sometimes he was irritable and moodier than usual; other times he was bothered by thoughts of ending his life even though he was a religious man and these thoughts shocked him.

Doug agreed to a SPECT scan, and not surprisingly he had markedly increased activity in his limbic system and an area of decreased activity in his left prefrontal cortex and left temporal lobe that likely were areas injured in his accident. These abnormalities were likely responsible for the headaches, suicidal thoughts, nausea, visual changes, and irritability Doug was experiencing.

Like most Type 6 patients, Doug responded well to the combination of an anticonvulsant and an antidepressant. Since he had a history of head injury and a current depression, we chose Lamictal for its low side-effect pro-

Doug's Before and After Treatment with Lamictal/Effexor

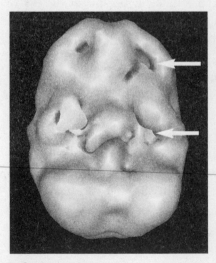 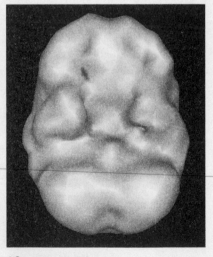

Before treatment
Underside surface view
Decreased left prefrontal cortex activity
(top arrow) and decreased left
temporal lobe activity (bottom arrow).

After treatment
Underside surface view
Overall improved activity.

file and antidepressant qualities. After Doug was no longer experiencing the headaches, suicidal thoughts, and irritability, we added Effexor to further treat his depression.

Type 7: Unfocused Anxiety/Depression—Low Prefrontal Cortex or Overall Brain Activity and a Hot BG and/or DLS

Type 7, Unfocused Anxiety/Depression is another variant for which a person often requires a combination of medications to reach the goal of maximizing brain performance. The core symptoms of anxiety and depression require treatment with one or more of the interventions specific to those disorders. However, the person with Type 7 is struggling with another complicating factor that must be addressed in order to optimize outcome. Type 7 people have low prefrontal cortex activity that does not improve with concentration. This is different from the pattern we see on SPECT scans of other types of depressed and anxious patients.

Typically, people with depression have normal prefrontal cortex function or alternatively may have decreased activity on their baseline SPECT scans. When they concentrate, the activity level in their prefrontal cortex improves. People with Unfocused Anxiety and/or Depression show a different pattern. Their prefrontal cortex has decreased function at baseline that does not improve with concentration. The inability of their prefrontal cortex to activate with concentration accounts for their complaints of inability to concentrate, poor decision making, lack of focus, distractibility, impulsivity, and disorganization. This area of the brain also helps modulate energy levels, goal setting, and many aspects of personality functioning. This pattern of deactivation that does not improve with concentration may be limited to the prefrontal cortex or may involve the brain in general.

Since we have made the decision to treat Type 7 with a combination of medications, deciding which medications to use requires identifying and prioritizing target symptoms so that one medication may be started at a time. Some case examples may be the best way to illustrate this point.

Rae Ann, twenty-seven, was having trouble with her memory, and even though she knew it was "almost impossible to have Alzheimer's disease so young," she seemed to be making more mistakes than usual and this was causing her trouble at work. She misplaced things, her attention span seemed short, and she couldn't concentrate. Rae Ann's memory problems started after she had been feeling sad for several weeks. She had been unable to sleep through the night for over a month, felt exhausted during the day, and wanted to take naps. She had no appetite and nothing seemed important to her anymore.

Rae Ann had tried increasing her time at the gym in the hope of feeling better but that only caused more fatigue. She had never used much alcohol but had given that up, too, by the time she came to the clinic. Her SPECT studies showed increased activity in her limbic system on both baseline and concentration scans. She also had decreased activity in her prefrontal cortex on her baseline scan that worsened with concentration.

Rae Ann had Type 7, Unfocused Depression and was initially started on Wellbutrin. We recommended this antidepressant for her because it treats depression and often helps mild prefrontal cortex symptoms. Rae Ann had a good antidepressant response to Wellbutrin, and, since her prefrontal cortex symptoms were not fully controlled on the antidepressant alone, we added a stimulant. Rae Ann then experienced full remission of her symptoms.

Dale decided his last trip to the emergency room was also "the last straw." This successful forty-nine-year-old businessman and father of four had been struggling with another bout of panic attacks. They seemed to come at the absolutely most inconvenient times and they scared him almost to death. Again and again Dale had gone to the local emergency room, sure he was having a heart attack, and each time the doctors had checked him out and told him it was "anxiety."

Dale was also more irritable than usual. His efficiency level and performance weren't what they used to be and his business was suffering because of it. The more aggravated Dale became with himself, the more difficulty he had concentrating. He misplaced things, too. Finding his car keys in the morning was a major undertaking and the process upset the entire family. Dale wondered if his marriage would survive if something wasn't done soon.

Dale's SPECT series showed markedly increased activity in his basal ganglia and decreased activity of his prefrontal cortex on baseline scan. Dale's basal ganglia remained overactive on his concentration scan and the activity level of his prefrontal cortex did not improve. Dale's history and scan findings show that he had Type 7, Unfocused Anxiety, and because his basal ganglia were so active we recommended treatment with an anticonvulsant as the first step. When Dale was no longer experiencing panic and anxiety, we added a stimulant to increase the performance of his prefrontal cortex. The stimulant further reduced Dale's difficulty with concentration, procrastination, and misplacing objects, and improved his attention span. If we had started the stimulant first, Dale's anxiety level would likely have increased because stimulants frequently cause a temporary increase in energy levels and agitation.

Stimulants are traditionally used to treat ADD in children and adults. Our current understanding of how stimulants work is that they increase dopamine output from the basal ganglia and increase activity in the prefrontal cortex and temporal lobes. The following tables summarize information about the most commonly used stimulant and non-stimulant medications presently available.

Contrary to popular belief, stimulants are very safe medications. The PDR lists 60mg as the top dosage for Ritalin, and 40mg as the top dosage

Stimulants				
Generic name	Brand name	Milligrams a day/ Available strengths	Times a day	Notes
amphetamine salt combination	Adderall (sustained release)	5 to 80/ 5, 7.5, 10, 12.5, 15, 20, 30	1 to 2	Adderall is long-acting and wears off smoothly. Also, the tablets are double scored. This makes it easy to quarter them and fine-tune the dose.
methylphenidate	Ritalin	5 to 120/ 5, 10, 20	2 to 4	Watch for rebound when it wears off.
methylphenidate HCl	Methylin (immediate and sustained release)	5 to 120/ 5, 10, 20	2 to 4	Watch for rebound when immediate release wears off.
methylphenidate sustained release	Ritalin SR (sustained release)	10 to 120/ 20	1 to 2	Many say it's erratic in its effect. We find that many doctors underdose it. It is only 50–60% bioavailable, which means you have to give more to get the same effect as regular Ritalin.

Generic name	Brand name	Milligrams a day/ Available strengths	Times a day	Notes
methylphen- idate HCl	Metadate ER and Metadate CD (sustained release)	10 to 120/ 10, 20	1 to 2	As above, may need higher doses to achieve best control of symptoms.
dextroam- phetamine	Dexedrine, Dextrostat	5 to 80/ 5, (10 generic only)	2 to 4	Watch for rebound when it wears off.
dextroam- phetamine slow-release caps	Dexedrine Spansules (sustained release)	5 to 80/ 5, 10, 15	1 to 2	Seems more reliable than Ritalin SR.
Pemoline	Cylert	18.75 to 112.5; up to 150 adults/ 18.75, 37.5, 75	1 to 2	Routine liver screen- ing is essential. Lasts longer than regular- release Ritalin or Dexedrine. We use Cylert last because of the liver toxicity issue.
methylphen- idate HCl	Concerta	18 to 54/ 18, 36, 54	1 to 2	The favorite of most doctors in our clinics. Can be dosed once daily, long-acting, smooth when wear- ing off, and very low side-effect profile.
dexmethyl- phenidate HCl	Focalin	5 to 20/ 2.5, 5, 10	1 to 2	A more active isomer of Ritalin. Short- acting for flexible dosing.

for Adderall and Dexedrine. Many clinicians, including the authors, feel the range of effectiveness may be much higher for some individuals. A study performed at Harvard indicated that adults, on average, need about 1 mil- ligram per kilogram of body weight per day. So if someone weighs 79 kilo-

Non-Stimulants				
Generic name	Brand name	Milligrams a day/ Available strengths	Times a day	Notes
atomoxetine	Straterra	For children—0.5 to 1.2 per kg of body weight. For adults 10 to 120/ 10, 18, 25, 40, 60	1 to 2	Newest non-stimulant medication approved for ADHD
modafinil (non-amphetamine stimulant)	Provigil	200/ 100, 200	1	Nonaddictive agent that improves alertness and increases wakefulness.
venlafaxine (antidepressant)	Effexor	37.5 to 375/ 25, 37.5, 50, 75, 100; and XR 37.5, 75, 150	1 to 2	Can increase blood pressure. Immediate release is taken twice daily, and XR is taken once daily. Should be tapered to avoid discontinuation syndrome.
*buproprion (antidepressant)	Wellbutrin	50 to 450/ 75, 100	1 to 2	Never give more than 150mg per dose. Do not exceed 450mg per day. Do not use in combination with other drugs that lower seizure threshold if the person is prone to seizures. Excellent for complaints of sexual dysfunction.
*buproprion sustained release (antidepressant)	Wellbutrin SR	150 to 450/ 100, 150	1 or 2	Never give more than 300mg a dose. Do not exceed 450mg per day. Do not use in combination with other drugs that lower seizure threshold if the person is prone to seizures.

*These medications are more fully discussed under the review of Type 2 earlier in this chapter.

Generic name	Brand name	Milligrams a day/ Available strengths	Times a day	Notes
*buproprion (continued)				Excellent for complaints of sexual dysfunction. The SR tablets should never be divided.
tranylcypro-mine sulfate MAOI	Parnate	30 to 60/ 10	2 to 3	Very potent drug that requires close moni-toring to avoid serious side effects due to dietary and drug-drug interactions. Also may help treatment-resistant anxiety disorders.
*imipramine TCA	Tofranil	10 to 300/ 10, 25, 50, 75, 100, 125	1 to 2	Also used to treat panic and other anxiety disorders. Helpful with bed-wetting.
*desipra-mine TCA	Norpramin	10 to 300/ 10, 25, 50, 75, 100, 150	1 to 2	Often helpful for several types of depressive disorders. Should be used with caution in children because of reports of sudden death.

*These medications are more fully discussed under the review of Type 2 earlier in this chapter.

grams (about 150 pounds), he will need an average dose of 70mg of stimulant a day. Because 2 to 3 percent of people taking Cylert develop a chemical hepatitis, it is very important to monitor the liver function of people taking this medication. For this reason, we usually reserve Cylert as the last choice.

It is essential to avoid taking stimulants with citrus juices (orange, grapefruit, lemon) or anything with citric acid in it (read labels, as citric acid is used in many things as a preservative) because it tends to lessen the effect of these medications. We also counsel our patients to decrease caffeine intake when they are taking a stimulant so as not to overstimulate the nervous system.

Combinations

Some people have symptoms that overlap categories. Others have symptoms that seem to fit into multiple categories. In these cases, a combination of medications might make the difference between a good response and an excellent response. As we studied thousands of brain scans we noticed that children of alcoholics often had brain patterns that responded to a combination of stimulants and anti-obsessional medications. We also realized that some people have multiple brain systems involved that need sophisticated combinations of medications to promote brain health.

We must stress once again that complex treatment plans that involve multiple medications require close supervision by a well-qualified specialist. It also means taking medications on a schedule, paying careful attention to diet and fitness, and informing all your doctors about every medication you take. You must also inform all your doctors of all over-the-counter medications, herbs, and supplements you take because these also interact with medications. It means decreasing caffeine and avoiding nicotine, drugs, and alcohol.

Remember
The goal needs to be the best functioning,
not to be off medication!

Many people mistakenly believe they can take only a "little bit" of the medication. This often causes the medication to be ineffective. The following metaphor illustrates how ill advised this practice is:

When a person goes to the eye doctor because she is having trouble seeing, she wants a prescription for glasses that will help her see the best. She doesn't ask for "just a little bit of a lens," she wants to see clearly!

So it is with anxiety and depression symptoms; everyone is different in the quantity of medication they require to function at their best. For some people, it is 5mg of medication one to two times a day. For others, it is much more. Everyone is different.

The side effects of not treating brain dysfunction are immeasurably worse than those caused by the medication!

CHAPTER 8

Natural Solutions:
Supplement Strategies
for the Seven Types

At least once a month a patient tells us about an amazing new treatment for anxiety or depression. Because we want to know about everything that works to help these disorders, we keep an open mind. Megavitamin therapy, herbs, fish oil, amino acids, and magnets are just a few examples of "miracle cures" that haven't been the panaceas predicted by the media hype. For many years we have followed alternative-medicine trends, reviewed the sparse scientific literature that exists, and evaluated the performance of many compounds to see what really works for our patients. Wading through the often-exaggerated claims and witnessing the initial excitement and later disappointment of patients at the all too familiar failure of "natural" treatments to deliver what they promise is challenging. We continue to meet this challenge, though, because we have found several alternative and complementary medicine interventions to be of great benefit to our patients when correctly matched to the type of disorder and the severity of symptoms.

People often believe that anything labeled "natural," "herbal," "organic," or "derived entirely from plant sources" can do no harm. This is absolutely untrue. Naturopathic, alternative, Asian, or herbal remedies have every potential to cause the serious consequences that people fear with standard drugs. Naturopathic compounds can trigger allergic reactions, interact with other drugs and supplements in toxic ways, and interfere with the action of birth control pills, and they have been known to cause death. Not all of these substances are innocuous or innocent compounds. Kava kava, for instance, has been removed from European markets because of its link to liver failure. And, in Japan, *sho-saikoto,* a previously very popular naturopathic intervention containing licorice and ginger root, thought to delay the onset of liver cancer after hepatitis C infection, has come under fire for its association with severe pneumonia and death. Clearly, "natural" doesn't always mean without consequences.

Modern pharmaceuticals have their roots in nature. Almost everyone knows that penicillin, the mother of our antibiotic industry, originally came from mold. Aspirin came from a plant source, as did the powerful heartbeat stabilizer digitalis. The original antimalarial drug, quinine, came from the bark of a South American tree, and now that most malaria is resistant to the old drugs, the new ones are derived from another plant source—the sweet woodworm plant in China. So, whether you choose alternative medicine or standard pharmaceuticals, you can feel confident that your choice has its roots in nature.

We have found that there are supplements that are beneficial to our patients with each type of anxiety and depression. Because of the lack of standardization among alternative treatments there are many different doses often recommended for any particular compound. The doses and the dosing schedules we provide are the ones that we have found to be most helpful without creating significant side effects for the majority of our patients.

We treat some patients with alternative medicine as the only medical intervention for their symptoms. Some of these patients come to us wanting to "try alternative medicine first to see if it works" before taking a standard medication. We treat others who cannot tolerate conventional medications because of side effects or allergies with alternative interventions. In many cases, we add supplements to standard drug therapy to boost its effectiveness. Additionally, there are some compounds we firmly believe are beneficial to everyone, regardless of health status. When we recommend alternative medicine and supplements to our patients we begin with a discussion about what is known about how these compounds work, the best dosage, how and when to take them, the expected side effects, and what to do if this option fails.

Most of the information we have about alternative medicine is not derived from scientific study, but rather from less rigorous tests of effectiveness and what we call "subjective reports." Subjective data are based entirely on a patient's personal experience or interpretation of how a product makes them feel. What they report may or may not be in agreement with what a scientist observes. Supplements and alternative medicines are not controlled by the FDA like conventional drugs and therefore can vary widely in the amount of active compound they contain. Pesticides or heavy metals may contaminate some foreign sources of herbal compounds.

Patients need to take alternative medications and supplements with the same seriousness that they do conventional medications. These compounds must be taken as prescribed, in the appropriate dose, and for the correct problem—otherwise, they won't work and in some cases might even make things worse.

Seventeen-year-old Josh was brought to see us by his mother. He had symptoms of anxiety and depression, along with periods of anger and moodiness. Several months before we met Josh, his mother had read a magazine article about St. John's wort that said that the drug helps with mood and temper problems, and she gave it to her son. Within a week Josh's behavior deteriorated. He was angrier and more agitated, and he started to have violent dreams. Josh's symptoms improved when his mother stopped giving him St. John's wort. As part of Josh's evaluation at our clinic, we did a SPECT scan that showed decreased activity in his left temporal lobe (Temporal Lobe Anxiety/Depression). Josh had one of the brain patterns that we have discovered is often made worse by serotonergic drugs, and St. John's wort is one of these drugs. Josh needed an anticonvulsant medication immediately to improve the function of his temporal lobe and to decrease his moodiness and anger. Once these behaviors stabilized, an antidepressant could be added. Later, he had a very positive response to Neurontin and Effexor.

Our patients are always counseled to keep a simple medication diary when they are starting new interventions. We ask them to record when they take supplements, medications, and other compounds; any side effects; and any changes in their symptoms. It is very important that patients always inform their doctors of all supplements, vitamins, medications, and naturopathic remedies they are taking. Many of these substances can interfere with the action of other medications, can produce side effects on their own, or can reach toxic levels if used inappropriately.

Supplements for the Seven Types

100 Percent Multivitamin and Mineral Supplement

We believe you should take a multivitamin and mineral supplement every day regardless of the type of anxiety or depression you have. In fact, you should take a multivitamin even if you are perfectly healthy and don't have anxiety or depression of any sort. We were taught in medical school that people who eat a balanced diet do not need supplemental vitamins or minerals, but this is simply not true for many people. The nutritional needs of a large number of the population are not being met because of their reliance on fast food. The elderly need supplementation, as they frequently do not eat well because of income limitations, difficulty preparing food, or lack of interest in eating. Adult women rarely get enough iron, calcium, and protein in their diets and benefit from a multivitamin.

In our experience, anxiety and depression compound the problem of meal planning. Families afflicted with anxiety and/or depression tend to eat out more frequently than other families because they are unable to execute all the steps necessary to arrange for meals. Protect yourself and your child by taking a 100 percent vitamin and mineral supplement.

Antioxidant Vitamins

All vitamins and minerals are not created equally. Some forms and preparations are more biologically active and available than others. The most expensive brands are not always the best; however, good products from reliable companies usually cost more than products that may not be absorbed in your system after you take them. There are many reputable manufacturers of vitamins and supplements, including TwinLab and Schiff, and patients should thoroughly investigate the brand they choose. An excellent resource for evaluating a particular brand of vitamin or herbal supplement is *www. consumerlab.com*.

Vitamin C has many powerful benefits. It is an antioxidant; it bolsters the immune system; and it is necessary for healthy connective tissue, tendons, and ligaments. The antioxidant effects of vitamin C protect brain and heart function. Five hundred to 1000mg should be taken two to three times every day. If you take a stimulant, you need to take vitamin C one hour before or two hours after your stimulant because it may interfere with absorption.

Vitamin E is a fat-soluble vitamin that protects cells from free radicals and other by-products of metabolism and stress. This antioxidant vitamin strengthens the immune system and may play a role in decreasing the risk or delaying the onset of some cancers. Vitamin E should be taken twice daily in doses of 400 to 600 IU. The natural *d*-alpha-tocopherol form is the best vitamin E preparation.

Anti-inflammatory Medications

Ibuprofen, an anti-inflammatory pain medication, has been shown in several studies to enhance memory and perhaps delay the onset of Alzheimer's disease. It probably works by decreasing inflammation in the brain and allowing better circulation. A dose of 200mg taken once a day with food is recommended. The cyclooxygenase inhibitor Vioxx appears to be even more effective but the cost is a limiting factor for most people.

Supplements for Type 1, Pure Anxiety

The supplements we recommend for Type 1, Pure Anxiety patients are those that act on the basal ganglia to calm brain activity.

Gamma-aminobutyric acid (GABA) is an amino acid that also functions as a neurotransmitter in the brain. In the herbal literature, GABA is reported to work in much the same way as the anti-anxiety and anticonvulsant drugs. It helps stabilize nerve cells by decreasing their tendency to fire erratically or excessively. This means it has a calming effect for people who struggle with temper, irritability, and anxiety, whether these symptoms relate to anxiety or to temporal lobe disturbance. GABA can be taken as a supplement in doses ranging from 250 to 1,500mg daily for adults, and from 125 to 750mg daily for children. For best effect, GABA should be taken in two to three divided doses.

Ruth came to see us for anxiety and irritability. She said her husband was very upset with her because she snapped angrily at him and the children on a regular basis. She had suffered from nervousness and feelings of panic ever since she could remember. She usually felt on edge, keyed up, and tense. In addition, she suffered from headaches and an upset stomach. Her mother had a Valium addiction, and Ruth wanted to avoid prescription medication for fear of addiction and side effects. Her SPECT scan showed excessive activity in the basal ganglia. We put her on GABA, at doses of 250mg three times a day. Within two weeks she reported that she felt calmer and more under control, and that her headaches and upset stomach were much better. In addition to the GABA, she was taught in therapy to deal with negative thoughts and to do relaxation exercises.

Ruth's Before and After Treatment with GABA

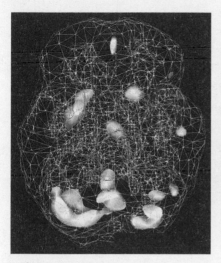 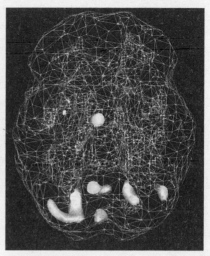

Before treatment
Increased basal ganglia activity.

After treatment
Overall calming of basal ganglia activity.

Vitamin B-6 (pyridoxine) and L-glutamine

Vitamin B-6 supports the action of the enzymes that convert the amino acid L-glutamine to GABA in the brain. Anxious people may not have enough L-glutamine or they may have vitamin B-6 deficiencies, which render them deficient in the building blocks necessary for GABA production. GABA is one of the amino acid–based neurotransmitters with inhibitory properties and decreases the rate of nerve cell firing. We recommend 500mg of glutamine three to four times daily between meals, and 50 to 100mg of vitamin B-6 twice daily. A cautionary note: Excessive doses of vitamin B-6 may cause nerve damage that is usually reversible when vitamin B-6 is stopped.

Kava

While we continue to get inquiries about kava kava, we have been suspicious of this compound for some time now and no longer recommend its use. It was recently withdrawn from some of the European markets because of its association with liver failure. Kava kava was previously recommended by some alternative-medicine practitioners to calm anxiety, promote healthy sleep, and reduce the physical and emotional effects of stress. Kava is thought to work by enhancing the production of GABA in the brain. It comes from the root of a South Pacific pepper tree and is widely used as a social and ceremonial drink in the Pacific Islands. The herb is so widely used that it is thought to be responsible, in part, for the laid-back lifestyle of the "islands." Kava has known interactions with alcohol, barbiturates, MAOIs, benzodiazepines, other tranquilizers and sleeping pills, anticoagulants, antiplatelet agents, including aspirin, antipsychotics, drugs used for treating Parkinson's disease, and drugs that suppress the central nervous system. Kava can exacerbate Parkinson's disease and increase muscle weakness and twitching. Women who are pregnant or breast-feeding should not take kava. We believe this supplement has more side effects and potential dangerous outcomes than benefits.

Valerian

Many of our patients find valerian to be remarkably helpful as a sleeping aid. Valerian is a well-recognized herb with anti-anxiety properties that is used as a mild tranquilizer, sedative, and muscle relaxant. There are about 150 species of valerian widely distributed in temperate regions of the world. The active ingredient is found in a foul-smelling oil produced in the root of the plant. The Roman physician Galen wrote about the virtues of valerian. It has been associated with the term "All Heal" in medical literature of the Middle Ages and is also used in Chinese and Indian medicine. It was used in the United States prior to the development of modern pharmaceuticals. This centuries-old treatment for insomnia has also been helpful to treat symptoms of nervousness, stress, increased emotional reactivity, pain, and agitation and to decrease seizure frequency for epileptic patients. Valerian appears to work by enhancing the activity of the calming neurotransmitter GABA. Studies have shown valerian to be helpful for many types of anxiety disorders and for people with performance anxiety and those who get stressed in daily situations, such as traffic. Valerian is available in capsules, tablets, liquids, tinctures, extracts, and teas. Most extracts are standardized to 0.8 percent valeric acids. Unlike prescription tranquilizers, valerian has a much lower potential for addiction and has been used to help people who are trying to decrease their use of prescription tranquilizers or sleeping pills. Anyone using prescription sleeping pills or tranquilizers should decrease or stop their use only under the supervision of a physician. Sometimes valerian can cause nervousness or drowsiness; make sure you know how your body reacts to it before you drive or do other activities that require sustained attention. Do not take valerian with alcohol, barbiturates, or benzodiazepines. Valerian is not recommended for use during pregnancy or breast-feeding. The recommended dose of valerian is 150 to 450mg in capsules or teas.

Phil, a forty-two-year-old chiropractor, came to see us for insomnia and anxiety. He said that he felt tense and keyed up most days and his anxiety prevented him from getting good, consistent sleep. He had tried numerous behavioral interventions without success. His anxiety interfered with his work performance, as he often appeared stressed to his patients. He was opposed to trying medication and wanted a recommendation for a natural treatment. GABA was ineffective for Phil, so we suggested 150mg of valerian in the morning and 300mg at night. Over the next several weeks he noticed that he felt more relaxed during the day and slept much better at night. He took valerian for six months and then slowly tapered and stopped it. He was then better able to use behavioral interventions to control his anxiety.

Supplements for Type 2, Pure Depression

This type of depression is most likely related to deficiencies in the neurotransmitters norepinephrine and dopamine. The supplements that most often help this type are DL-phenylalanine (DLPA), L-tyrosine, and S-Adenosyl-Methionine (SAMe).

DLPA is the amino acid precursor for norepinephrine. A number of studies show norepinephrine and epinephrine (adrenaline) is low in patients with depression. The antidepressants imipramine and desipramine work by increasing norepinephrine in the brain. Theoretically, when more precursor is available, more neurotransmitter will be made. Therefore it makes sense that, by boosting DLPA, we can increase norepinephrine and have a positive impact on mood. In fact, in a number of studies DLPA has been found to be helpful for depression, energy, and pain control. Dr. Amen has used it for fifteen years as an antidepressant in children, teens, and adults. It is milder in its effect than prescribed antidepressants, but it causes significantly fewer side effects. People who have PKU (phenylketonuria) should not take DLPA because they do not have the enzyme that metabolizes it. DLPA is recommended in doses of 400mg three times a day on an empty stomach for adults, and 20mg three times daily for children.

Brian, a fifteen-year-old high school student, came to see us at his own request. He said that he often felt negative and had too many negative thoughts, and he was often tired. He didn't want to take medication and wanted to know if there were "natural things" he could do. We had him exercise, eat a more balanced diet, and take 400mg of DLPA three times a day on an empty stomach. Within two weeks he said he felt much better and was more focused, more energetic, and more positive. He recently wrote us from college saying he has remained faithful to his regimen and continues to feel well four years later.

L-tyrosine is an amino acid building block for dopamine, epinephrine, and norepinephrine. It helps to boost energy levels, mood, and metabolism. L-tyrosine may increase motivation and improve concentration. We recommend L-tyrosine in doses of 100 to 500mg two to three times daily for children under twelve, and 500 to 1,500mg two to three times daily for adults. The first dose should be taken in the morning on an empty stomach and the other doses should be taken between meals. Patients with Type 4, Overfocused Anxiety/Depression may experience an increase in symptoms of obsessiveness and irritability with L-tyrosine and should start with low doses. Patients with a history of mania should exercise caution with the use of L-tyrosine because its energizing properties may trigger a manic episode. The side effects we see with DLPA and L-tyrosine in our practice are limited to mild weight loss.

Michael, forty, had been treated for depression for several years and could not seem to stay well. It seemed that, no matter which medication Michael tried, it worked for a while and then, maddeningly, the effectiveness wore off and Michael's symptoms returned. The off-and-on-again usefulness of the medications was extremely frustrating for Michael. He was ready for something different. We recommended 1,000mg of L-tyrosine three times daily, firm adherence to a new diet, and fast walking five times a week as a fitness goal. Michael was intensely committed to his new program and felt better within a week. Anyone who has ever tried medication knows this is a very rapid response. He has maintained his feeling of well-being for three years now.

SAMe is involved with the production of several neurotransmitters. The brain normally manufactures all the SAMe it needs from the amino acid methionine. When a person is depressed, the synthesis of SAMe from methionine is impaired. SAMe is one of the best natural antidepressants, and in a number of recent studies it has performed as well as conventional antidepressant medications. SAMe has been found to increase the neurotransmitters that are low when people have depression. We frequently recommend

SAMe to people who suffer from fibromyalgia, a chronic muscle pain disorder. Fibromyalgia is very commonly complicated by anxiety and depression. *People who have Bipolar Disorder or manic-depressive illness should not take SAMe.* There have been a number of reported cases of SAMe causing manic or hypomanic episodes (excessively up or happy moods, extreme impulsivity in sexuality or spending money, pressured speech, and decreased need for sleep). SAMe should be taken in doses of 200 to 400mg two to four times a day; children should take half this amount. One of the problems with SAMe is its cost. It is as expensive as many of the newer antidepressants and insurance companies do not cover herbal or supplemental treatments, which makes SAMe more expensive than prescription medication for most people. As it becomes a more popular intervention, the cost of SAMe may decrease.

Ted was forty-two when his wife insisted that he see us. He was negative, irritable, and lethargic. Ted battled constantly with the children, bickered with his wife, and had no interest in sex. He had significant arthritic pain, which made him even more irritable and cranky. His SPECT study showed markedly increased activity in his limbic system. We started him on 400mg of SAMe twice a day. Within three weeks Ted was feeling better, and he had more energy and was in less pain. His wife and children all noticed a positive difference in his interactions with them.

Supplements for Type 3, Mixed Anxiety/Depression

This type of anxiety and/or depression often needs a combination of Pure Anxiety and Pure Depression supplements. We find that a combination of SAMe and GABA is often helpful for our patients with Mixed Anxiety/Depression.

Supplements for Type 4, Overfocused Anxiety/Depression

Patients with Overfocused Anxiety/Depression most likely have a relative deficiency of the neurotransmitter serotonin. We have seen dramatic improvement in many of our patients on St. John's wort and have SPECT scan studies of patients before and after treatment with St. John's wort that document its effectiveness. This flowering herb is named after St. John the Baptist because it blooms around June 24, his feast day, and because the red ring around the crushed flowers is a reminder of the blood of the beheaded saint. St. John's wort may be the most potent of all the supplements at increasing serotonin availability in the brain. The starting dosage of St. John's wort is 300mg a day for children, 300mg twice a day for teens, and 600mg in the morning and 300mg at night for adults. Sometimes the dose may be increased slowly to 1,800mg for adults. It is extremely important that the preparation of St. John's wort contains 0.3 percent hypericin, which is believed to be the active ingredient. St. John's wort decreases anterior cingulate gyrus hyperactivity for many patients and decreases moodiness. An unfortunate side effect is that it can decrease prefrontal cortex activity. One of the women in the study said, "I'm happier, but I'm dingier." St. John's wort may make people more vulnerable to sunburn, so extra sun protection is needed by anyone using this compound. We also don't start people with temporal lobe symptoms (anger, epilepsy, memory problems, hallucinations, and so on) on St. John's wort without first stabilizing the temporal lobes with anticonvulsant medication.

Allie, thirteen, had always been a worrier. When things didn't go her way at home, she had temper outbursts. She worried about her grades and

Allie's Before and After Treatment with St. John's wort

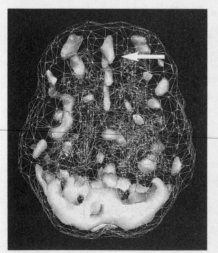 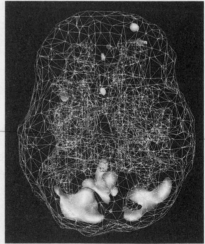

Before treatment
Increased anterior cingulate gyrus activity (arrow).

After treatment
Overall calming of anterior cingulate gyrus activity.

spent excessive time on assignments. Her mother, a school administrator, brought her to the Amen Clinic after she heard one of our lectures. She said she was sure Allie had an overactive cingulate gyrus. Allie's SPECT study confirmed her mother's suspicions. Within a month on St. John's wort, Allie felt better. She was more relaxed, less upset over disappointments, and she spent less time obsessing over her schoolwork.

Serotonin Pathway

Tryptophan

↓

5-HTP

↓

Serotonin

↓

N-acetyl-serotonin

↓

Melatonin

L–tryptophan and 5–HTP are amino acid building blocks for serotonin and taking these supplements can increase cerebral serotonin. L–tryptophan is a naturally occurring amino acid found in milk, meat, and eggs. It is very helpful for some patients in improving sleep, decreasing aggressiveness, and stabilizing mood. It does not have side effects and this is a real advantage over prescription antidepressants. L–tryptophan was taken off the market a number of years ago because one contaminated batch, from one manufacturer, caused a rare blood disease and a number of deaths. L–tryptophan itself actually had nothing to do with the deaths. L–tryptophan was recently reapproved by the Food and Drug Administration and is now available by prescription. One of the problems with dietary L–tryptophan is that a significant portion of it does not enter the brain but is used to make proteins and vitamin B–3. This necessitates taking large amounts of tryptophan. Recommended dosage is 1,000 to 3,000mg at bedtime.

5–HTP is a step closer in the serotonin production pathway. It is also more widely available than L–tryptophan and is more easily taken up in the brain. Seventy percent is taken up into the brain, as opposed to only 3 percent of L-tryptophan. 5-HTP is about five to ten times more powerful than L-tryptophan. A number of double-blind studies have shown 5-HTP to be an effective antidepressant medication that is relatively free of the side effects caused by conventional medications. Decreased serotonin levels in the brain have been correlated with depression, aggressive feelings, and violence. 5-HTP boosts serotonin levels in the brain and helps to calm anterior cingulate gyrus hyperactivity. This is analogous to greasing (increasing serotonin) the brain's gear shifter (anterior cingulate gyrus) so that attention, focus, and concentration can be locked into place and yet also smoothly and efficiently shifted on to the next item when necessary. Adults should take 5-HTP in doses of 50 to 100mg two to three times daily with or without food, and children should take half the adult dose. Many alternative-medicine doctors believe patients who are taking 5-HTP should also take vitamin B-6, 50mg once daily, because this vitamin is essential for converting amino acids into serotonin. The most common side effect of 5-HTP is an upset stomach, although this is usually a mild complaint. Upset stomach can be improved by starting 5-HTP slowly and increasing the dose as you get used to the supplement and by taking it with food. Because 5-HTP increases serotonin, you should not take other medications that also increase serotonin, such as St. John's wort, L-tryptophan, or prescribed antidepressants, unless you are closely supervised by your physician.

Supplements for Type 5,
Cyclic Anxiety/Depression

The supplements that our Type 5 patients have most benefited from are GABA, taurine, and fish oils. GABA, which is discussed under Type 1 and again under Type 6, is effective for Cyclic Anxiety/Depression because of its calming effect on nerve cells. This nerve cell stabilizing effect acts on the focal hyperactivity in the brain's limbic system that produces the symptoms of Cyclic Anxiety/Depression.

Taurine

Taurine is an inhibitory neurotransmitter, which stimulates the neurotransmitter GABA. It has a calming effect on the nervous system. Women in particular need to ingest enough taurine because estrogen depresses the formation of taurine in the liver. Women who use estrogen supplementation may need even more taurine. Alcohol increases the excretion of taurine in the urine, effectively depleting it from the body. Taurine is present in animal protein but not vegetable proteins, so vegetarians need to make sure they get enough. The recommended dose of taurine is 50mg a day. Taurine can be irritating to the stomach and may cause nausea at higher doses. People who have ulcer disease should avoid it.

Fish Oils

Supplementation with fish oils containing high levels of omega-3 fatty acids is also often helpful. An insufficiency of omega-3 fatty acids has been linked to depression and mood instability. This may be related to how fatty acids make up nerve cell membranes. Without high levels of omega-3 fatty acids, the nerve cell membranes are less fluid and may cause nerve cells to react sluggishly and misfire. Population-based studies in various countries, including the United States, have indicated increased rates of depression along with deteriorating dietary habits. Many social, educational, and neuroscientists are studying links between medical and neuropsychiatric illness and nutrient-poor diets. The decreased consumption of omega-3 fatty acids, quality proteins, essential vitamins, minerals, and even uncontaminated water may correlate with the skyrocketing rate of anxiety and depression. Omega-3 fatty acids are essential to good brain health. In a study done at Harvard and reported in the *Archives of General Psychiatry*, supplementation with high-dose purified fish oils provided a statistically significant improvement in Bipolar Disorder. Here are four ways to boost the level of omega-3 fatty acids in your diet:

1. Eliminate transfatty acids by avoiding margarine, shortening, and most processed foods.

2. Increase the consumption of tuna and cold-water fish, such as salmon, mackerel, herring, and halibut.

3. Take 1 tablespoon of flaxseed oil a day.

4. Eat Coromega, which is available at health food stores. It's a creamy, orange pudding–flavored preparation that is not oily, and kids like it because it does not cause "fish burps."

Supplements for Type 6,
Temporal Lobe Anxiety/Depression

Patients with Type 6, Temporal Lobe Anxiety/Depression and patients with temporal lobe epilepsy have symptoms that originate in the same area of the brain, which is why we often treat both of these groups with antiseizure or anticonvulsant medications. Stabilization and enhancement of temporal lobe function are the treatment goals for Type 6. Anticonvulsant medications work, at least in part, by enhancing the action of GABA. GABA is what we call an inhibitory neurotransmitter in the brain, and this means it decreases nerve cell activity by calming down their firing rate. GABA keeps nerve cells from overfiring or firing erratically and, in doing so, acts as an anticonvulsant.

Another benefit of GABA supplementation is its anti-anxiety effects. Many individuals who have temporal lobe symptoms also struggle with temper control, irritability, and anxiety, and GABA produces a calming effect in these cases. The alternative-medicine literature theorizes that GABA works in much the same way as minor tranquilizers such as Valium and Librium but does not cause addiction.

GABA can be taken as a supplement in doses of 250 to 500mg two to three times daily for a maximum daily dose of 1,500mg. Children usually take half the adult dose.

Many people with temporal lobe problems suffer from memory problems. We have found a number of natural substances helpful for memory enhancement, including:

- Phosphatidyl serine (PS): PS plays a major role in determining the integrity and fluidity of brain cell membranes. Except in cases of folic acid, vitamin B12, or essential fatty acid deficiency, the brain manufactures enough PS. Low levels of PS are associated with memory problems and depression in the elderly. There are eighteen double-blind studies supporting the effectiveness of PS supplementation for memory issue complaints. In the largest study, 494 elderly patients (ages sixty-five to ninety-three) with moderate to severe senility were given PS (100mg three times a day) or a placebo for six months. The patients were assessed for cognitive function, behavior, and mood at the beginning and end of the study. At the end of the study, patients who took PS showed statistically significant improvements in all three areas. The recommended dose of PS is 100mg twice a day for two weeks; then, if needed, 100mg three times a day for memory.

- Gingko biloba, from gingko trees, is a powerful antioxidant that is best known for its ability to enhance circulation. In a number of studies at major universities, gingko biloba has been shown to improve energy, concentration, focus, and memory. Gingko biloba has been reported to enhance cerebral blood flow and reduce or slow the symptoms of Alzheimer's disease. There are many different forms of gingko, making dosing confusing. Ginkoba and Ginkgold (Nature's Way) are brands that have been compounded to most resemble the compounds used in the major studies on gingko biloba. The recommended dose of gingko is 60 to 120mg twice a day.

Supplements for Type 7,
Unfocused Anxiety/Depression

This type is complicated by low prefrontal cortex or overall brain activity, as well as overactivity in the basal ganglia and deep limbic system. Strategies geared toward enhancing overall brain activity seem to be the most helpful. We especially like using supplements that enhance dopamine and norepinephrine, such as L-tyrosine, SAMe, and DLPA. We would also add fish oil to this combination to boost cellular transmission. Please refer to the sections above for a discussion of these compounds.

CHAPTER 9

Food Is a Drug: Dietary
Interventions for the Seven Types

Food is a drug. Food has powerful effects on cognition, feelings, and behavior. What you choose to eat changes how you feel about yourself, influences your mood, causes major changes in your general health and fitness level, and can make you crave more or swear off something forever. Diet and exercise are cornerstones of our treatment plans for patients with depression and anxiety. The right diet and fitness program can actually change the amount and/or type of medication a person needs. The wrong diet and lack of exercise can have the opposite effect.

Eating well does not mean sacrificing pleasure and it does not mean you need to become a slave to calorie counting and weighing and measuring complicated ratios of food portions. It means understanding your nutritional and fitness goals, reducing your risk of disease by increasing essential nutrients in your diet, and upgrading the quality of your dietary intake.

Unlike the conventional food pyramid, we look at food as falling into four groups: water, proteins, carbohydrates, and fats.

Water

The human body is two-thirds water. Water is an essential part of every function in the body, including blood flow to the brain and brain cell function. It helps transport nutrients and waste products in and out of cells. Without enough water the body becomes dehydrated and struggles to function properly. An abundance of water gives cells the opportunity to work well. Drink adequate amounts of water every day. Nutritionists recommend at least eight 8-ounce glasses a day. Avoid substances that dehydrate the body such as caffeine and alcohol, both of which cause increased urinary output.

Proteins

Proteins are essential to life. They are involved with immune system function, muscle mass, the enzymes that drive the chemical reactions of life, and hormones, and they are required for the manufacture of the neurotransmitters that make the brain function smoothly. Proteins are metabolized by the body into amino acids, the ultimate building blocks of the body's most important substances. There are two types of amino acids—essential and nonessential. The essential amino acids are those that must come from the diet. Nonessential amino acids are those that the body can manufacture for itself. There are two types of protein—complete and incomplete. Complete proteins are the best source of essential and nonessential amino acids. Complete proteins are found in meat, fish, poultry, cheese, eggs, yogurt, and soy products. Incomplete proteins have only some of the essential amino acids. They are found in a number of foods, such as grains, legumes, nuts, and leafy green vegetables.

Proteins are extremely important and breakfast is extremely important. In fact, we recommend that breakfast, for adults and children, include quality protein. Breakfast commonly consists of high-sugar, high-carbohydrate, low-protein, bad-for-your-brain cereal—especially for children. Carbohydrates are broken down in the body to sugar, and after the initial brief lift in energy that you feel, or increase in hyperactivity if you are an ADD child, you'll feel tired, cranky, and have trouble concentrating. Carbohydrates and sugars don't provide the dietary nutrients you need, and this means you're wasting your calories on them. Quality proteins throughout the day are necessary for brain and body health, weight management, hunger control, and to ensure adequate supplies of essential vitamins and nutrients.

High-quality Proteins

Chicken breast

Turkey breast

Shrimp, lobster, crab

Very lean cuts of beef, such as top sirloin and lean ground beef

Fish, especially salmon and tuna

Low-fat cottage cheese

Low-fat string cheese

Egg whites or egg substitutes

Protein shakes

A serving of protein is the size of your palm.

Carbohydrates

Carbohydrates come from plants and the fruit of trees. Milk and milk products are the only foods derived from animals that contain significant amounts of carbohydrates. There are three types of carbohydrates: sugar, simple carbohydrates, and complex carbohydrates. Sugar is a simple molecule that is used for energy and comes from several sources: fruit (fructose), sugarcane (sucrose), milk (lactose), corn (corn syrup), and glucose (sugar the body makes from dietary carbohydrate). When sugar or carbohydrate is consumed, it is rapidly absorbed into the bloodstream as glucose. High levels of blood glucose are sensed by the brain, which sets in motion a hormonal cascade to decrease the glucose level. The pancreas responds to signals from the pituitary gland and hypothalamus in the brain and releases insulin to drive glucose into the body's cells. Because the muscles and liver can store only a very small amount of glucose, the rest is stored as fat. As blood sugar levels fall, you feel tired and irritable and have trouble focusing. You may even start to feel hungry again, and if you happen to reach for a bagel, some chips, or candy, you will start the whole cycle over again.

Simple carbohydrates are sugar molecules connected by an oxygen molecule. They include pasta, bagels, bread, potatoes, rice, and cereals. They are very easily broken down to sugar in the stomach and rapidly enter the bloodstream, causing a rapid rise of blood sugar (notice how tired you feel after a spaghetti dinner). Complex carbohydrates, such as vegetables, whole grains, and beans, have more complex chemical bonds and take longer to be broken down in the stomach. They also have more fiber and water that help slow down the rate at which they are absorbed. In choosing carbohydrates for your or your child's diet, select complex carbohydrates such as fruits, vegetables, peas, beans, and whole grain products rather than sugar or simple carbohydrates. Complex carbohydrates are taken up in the bloodstream more slowly. Complex carbohydrates are less likely to cause an overproduction of insulin. In addition, they are filled with fiber, vitamins, and minerals— all essential ingredients to your health.

Quality Carbohydrates

Baked potatoes, no larger than your fist, topped with fat-free yogurt

Baked sweet potatoes, no larger than your fist, topped with fat-free yogurt

Whole wheat bread, one slice is one serving

Brown rice or wild rice, ½ cup is one serving

Oatmeal or grits, ½ cup is one serving

Pasta, whole wheat is best, ½ cup is one serving

Beans, ¼–½ cup is one serving

Leafy vegetables that go in salads can be eaten in any quantity; vinaigrettes should be used as dressings

Broccoli, green beans, peppers, tomatoes, onions, carrots, mushrooms, spinach, artichokes, celery, zucchini, cucumbers, cauliflower, ½ cup is one serving

Strawberries, melons, apples, oranges, grapefruits

Fats

Fat is the richest energy source. Dietary fat is essential during infancy and childhood for normal brain development. Fats come from both animal and plant sources and are composed of building blocks called fatty acids. The four types of fat in food are saturated, polyunsaturated, monounsaturated, and transfatty acids. During the last ten to fifteen years, there has been an increased effort on the part of nutritionists and the medical profession to raise public awareness about the dangers of dietary fats. An explosion of low-fat food products and dietary substitutes has deluged the market over the course of this time period and yet the rate of heart disease and obesity keeps increasing. Clearly, people are confused about which fats to cut out of their diet and what to replace them with.

Saturated fats and transfats are bad fats. These dietary fats are found in butter, cheese, whole milk, many animal products, chocolate, shortenings, and some oils such as coconut oil. These fats can increase your cholesterol level, which in turn increases your risk of heart disease and stroke. Polyunsaturated fats are in most vegetable oils and they tend to lower blood cholesterol levels. This may be deceiving, though, because they also undergo a metabolic event called oxidation, and this process can lead to an increase in plaque formation in the coronary arteries. Monounsaturated fats are decidedly the best fats. They may help lower blood cholesterol and they don't undergo oxidation. These fats are found in olive oil, canola oil, and nuts.

Bill Phillips, author of *Body for Life,* came up with one of the easiest ways to distinguish bad fats from good fats. He said, "If it is solid at room temperature, like butter, margarine, or shortening, it's bad news." In general, this is true and an easy rule to follow.

The brain is a unique organ in that more than half of its weight is composed of fat, nearly one-third of which is made up of the long-chain omega-3 fatty acid known as docosahexaenoic acid (DHA). This is an essential fatty acid, which means your body cannot manufacture it; you must get it from your diet. Omega-3 fatty acids are vital for the development of new neural pathways and for the maintenance of membrane fluidity at the neuronal synapse. This is a fancy way of saying that, without omega-3 fatty acids, your brain can't learn and it can't transmit signals. Rodent studies have proved that rats fed diets high in DHA have increased levels of both dopamine and serotonin in their frontal cortex compared to rats fed diets devoid of this fatty acid. Moreover, rats on the high-DHA diet had increased binding of dopamine to D2 brain receptors, and conversely, those with diets deficient in omega-3 fatty acids had a reduction of dopaminergic function. These changes in dopaminergic function correspond to the known adverse effects of omega-3 fatty acid deficiency on learning and the corresponding improvement of learning abilities with supplementation with fish oils that contain DHA.

Quality Fats

Olive oil

Canola oil

Avocados

Nuts, such as Brazil nuts, macadamia nuts, almonds, cashews, and pistachios

In using food as medicine, it is important to maintain a proper balance between proteins, carbohydrates, and fats.

Simple Steps to Dietary Success

1. Keep your metabolic rate at a constant level throughout the day by eating five meals a day. Breakfast is the most important meal. It starts your metabolism, blood flow, and energy tone for the day. Make sure you have some quality protein in the morning (such as lean meat, cottage cheese, eggs, nuts, or a protein shake). In fact, you should eat protein at every meal. Protein snacks are also important to help maintain good energy and concentration. Take sliced deli meats, low-fat yogurts, and cottage cheese to work with you to eat during the day. Protein contains the amino acid building blocks for neurotransmitters in the brain. Protein is essential to a "concentration diet."

2. Substitute complex carbohydrates (vegetables and whole grains) for the simple sugars and simple carbohydrates in your diet. Complex carbohydrates are broken down in the gut more slowly than simple carbohydrates. They also provide more fiber and nutrients. They still turn to glucose in your blood, so remember to eat their recommended serving portions. Some vegetables have a higher sugar content than others, so stick to our list under Quality Carbohydrates (page 177) when you begin your new lifestyle, and invest in some good reading material for additional help (see our Recommended Reading list).

3. Watch fruit and fruit juice intake. Most people think they can have an unlimited amount of fruit and fruit juices. Most fruits are very high in natural sugar (fructose), which can have the same effect on

blood sugar as sugar straight out of a box. Fruit is better than fruit juices because of the extra vitamins and fiber, but if you overconsume fruit you may feel sluggish and mentally slowed down. Fruits that tend to be especially good are apricots, oranges, tangerines, pears, grapefruit, apples, and kiwi. Avoid grapes, dates, and bananas because their sugar content seems to be the highest.

4. Eliminate most simple carbohydrates (this includes bread or pasta made with white flour; white rice; white potatoes; sugar; corn syrup; honey; and candy). A therapist told us this story at a recent lecture: "I'm so glad you mentioned sugar. I used to be a very angry person; sometimes I would even scare my family. It made me feel terrible. I took anger management classes, but they didn't seem to help. When I eliminated sugar from my diet, I noticed an almost immediate reduction in outbursts, plus I had better energy, lost weight, and was much more focused." His personal experience has been the same as our clinical experience.

5. Increase the amount of omega-3 fatty acids in your diet (large coldwater fish such as tuna and salmon, walnuts, Brazil nuts, and olive and canola oil). We review omega-3 fatty acids in more detail in the next chapter.

6. Do not get bored with your nutritional program. Invest in a couple of good cookbooks and dietary support guides that help you prepare good-tasting, high-quality meals. Take a look at *The Mayo Clinic Williams-Sonoma Cookbook* and the recipes in *Protein Power* (see our Recommended Reading list).

Here is a list of suggestions to help implement these dietary strategies.

Optimum Breakfast Options

Omelets with lean meats, low-fat cheese, or vegetables

Egg whites, egg substitutes

Turkey bacon and sausage

Cottage cheese and fruit

Cottage cheese and minute steak

Oatmeal (high in fiber and also contains gamma-linolenic acid, an essential fatty acid)

Protein shakes with a tablespoon of flaxseed oil (rich in omega-3 fatty acids) added

(Avoid sugar—sugar cereals, donuts, Pop-Tarts, waffles and pancakes with syrup, bagels, toast, cinnamon rolls)

Optimum Lunch Options

Stir-fry (vegetables and lean meat, no rice)

Cobb salad—no sugar in the dressing

Caesar salad with chicken breast (no sugar in the dressing, no croutons)

Tuna salad

Sandwiches made with lean protein and whole wheat bread

Sliced deli meats and raw sliced vegetables

Chicken breast (or any other lean meat), prepared any way except fried, and salad (use vinaigrette dressing)

Protein shake if you're really time-pressed

Boiled shrimp, and salad with vinaigrette dressing

Sandwich made with 100 percent natural peanut butter (Laura Scudder's makes a tasty brand) and 100 percent spreadable fruit jam (Smucker's makes sugar-free jam that tastes great—it's also a good topping on sugar-free ice cream)

(Avoid sugar and simple carbohydrates—white bread, french fries, breaded onion rings and meat, potato chips, ketchup, and potatoes—unless eaten with the skin)

Optimum Dinner Options

Salad

Lean protein—beef, chicken, pork, lamb, fish (highest in omega-3 fatty acids)

Vegetables

(Avoid sugar and simple carbohydrates—white bread, french fries, breaded onion rings and meat, potato chips, ketchup, and potatoes, unless eaten with the skin)

Snacks

Sugar-free ice cream

Cream cheese and celery

Raw or steamed vegetables

Low-fat cottage cheese

Apples

Strawberries

Melons

Oranges

Protein shakes

Olives

Sugar-free peanut butter and celery

Nuts, especially Brazil nuts (high in omega-3 fatty acids)

Homemade beef jerky—this is our personal favorite and we eat it all the time while writing. (Take flank steak and slice it thinly with the grain; put a little salt, pepper, and garlic powder on the meat and put it in a dehydrator. It's cheap, very tasty, and the kids like it a lot.)

Use these guidelines, especially when you or your child needs more energy, a more positive attitude, and mental clarity. These dietary guidelines will help you stabilize your blood sugar, lower your cholesterol, decrease your appetite, and lose weight. Your mood, ability to concentrate, and energy level will improve.

Overfocused Issues

Type 4, Overfocused Anxiety/Depression is often associated with worrying, moodiness, emotional rigidity, and irritability. A higher-protein, lower-carbohydrate diet (which enhances focus) may cause people with Over-focused Anxiety/Depression to focus more intently on negative thoughts or behaviors. Dietary interventions need to be geared toward naturally increasing serotonin, the neurotransmitter that is deficient in this type of anxiety and/or depression. The amino acid tryptophan is used to produce serotonin in the brain. Tryptophan is an essential amino acid and is found in abundance in all protein-rich foods, including dairy products, eggs, meat, fish, seeds, nuts, and a number of vegetables. Foods containing tryptophan also contain other amino acids. While it seems to be a reasonable assumption that a high-protein diet would increase serotonin levels, the opposite is true. When you eat a high-protein diet, tryptophan, which is a relatively small amino acid, does not compete well against the other amino acids and is actually lowered in the brain. Instead, it seems that carbohydrate-containing foods such as pasta, potatoes, bread, pastries, pretzels, candy, and popcorn actually increase L-tryptophan levels in the brain. In 1972 Dr. John Fern-strom and Dr. Richard Wurtman from MIT published their landmark study on carbohydrates and brain serotonin in the journal *Science*. The researchers showed that the protein and carbohydrate content of food has a significant impact on the production of serotonin. Cerebral serotonin and dopamine levels can be raised by eating a diet balanced between carbohydrates and protein. Many people unknowingly trigger cognitive inflexibility or mood problems by eating diets that are low in L-tryptophan. For example, high-protein, low-carbohydrate diets that we recommend for the other types of anxiety and depression increase dopamine and often make people with cingulate problems worse.

Pay attention to what you are eating as it will have an effect on your mood, attitude, and overall brain function.

CHAPTER 10

ANTs and ANTeaters: Cognitive Therapy for the Seven Types

Finally, brothers, whatever is true, whatever is noble, whatever is right, whatever is pure, whatever is lovely, whatever is admirable—if anything is excellent or praiseworthy—think about such things. Whatever you have learned or received or heard from me, or seen in me—put it into practice. And the God of peace will be with you.

LETTER FROM PAUL TO THE PHILIPPIANS, 4:8–9

Cognitive therapy, or therapy for your thoughts, has proven to be a very helpful tool in treating a wide variety of psychological problems—from depression and anxiety disorders to eating disorders and even marital or vocational problems. Most mental health professionals believe that either psychologist Albert Ellis or psychiatrist Aaron Beck invented cognitive therapy. That's true as far as twentieth-century psychology goes, yet it is clear in the Bible that the apostle Paul laid down the principles for cognitive therapy two thousand years before Ellis or Beck. Philippians 4:8–9 is a very clear statement on the most helpful way to think and behave. Paul understood the power of moment-by-moment thoughts on your life. What you allow to occupy your mind will sooner or later determine your feelings, your speech, and your actions.

Thoughts originate and become conscious through the release of chemicals and spreading electrical transmissions in your brain. Thoughts are biologically based and have a real impact on how you feel and behave. Every time you have an angry, unkind, sad, or cranky thought, your brain releases negative chemicals that activate your deep limbic system and make your body feel bad. Think about how you felt the last time you were mad. When most people are angry their muscles become tense, their hearts beat faster, their hands start to sweat, and they may even begin to feel a little dizzy.

Every time you have a good thought, a happy thought, a hopeful thought, or a kind thought, your brain releases chemicals that calm your deep limbic system and help your body feel good. Think about how you felt the last time you were happy. When most people are happy their muscles relax, their hearts beat slower, their hands become dry, and their breathing slows.

We can track the body's reaction to positive and negative stress from lie detector tests. During a lie detector test, a person is hooked up to equipment that measures hand temperature, heart rate, blood pressure, breathing rate, muscle tension, and how much the hands sweat. The tester then asks questions. If the person lies or tries to hide something, his body is likely to have a "stress" response and react in the following ways: hands get colder, heart beats more rapidly, blood pressure goes up, breathing quickens, muscles tighten, and hands sweat more. Almost immediately the subject's body reacts to his thoughts, whether or not he says anything. The deep limbic system is responsible for translating our emotional state into physical feelings of relaxation or tension. The opposite is also true. If he responds to a question truthfully, in all innocence, his body will likely experience a "relaxation" response and react in the following ways: hands become warmer, heart rate slows, blood pressure decreases, breathing slows and deepens, muscles relax, and hands become drier. No matter who you are, your body reacts to what you think. This not only happens when you're asked about telling the truth, your body reacts to every thought you have, whether it is about work, friends, family, or anything else.

Mark George, M.D., demonstrated the brain's reaction to thought in an elegant study of brain function at the National Institutes of Mental Health. He studied the activity of the brain in ten normal women under three different conditions: when they were thinking neutral thoughts, happy thoughts, and sad thoughts. During the neutral thoughts, nothing changed in the brain. During the happy thoughts, each woman demonstrated a cooling of her deep limbic system. During the sad thoughts, each woman's deep limbic system became highly active.

Thoughts are powerful. They can make your mind and your body feel good or they can make them feel bad. That is why emotional upset can manifest itself in physical symptoms such as headaches and stomachaches. Your body is like an ecosystem. An ecosystem contains everything in the environment, such as water, land, cars, people, animals, vegetation, houses, landfills, etc. A negative thought is like pollution to your system. Just as pollution in the Los Angeles Basin affects everyone who goes outside, so, too, do negative thoughts pollute your deep limbic system, your mind, and your body.

Thoughts are usually automatic but they are not necessarily correct, nor do they always tell the truth. In fact, they often lie. Most of us believe our thoughts and do not know how to challenge them or direct them in a helpful way.

The good news is that you can train your thoughts to be positive and hopeful or you can allow them to be negative and upset you. Once you are aware of what you can do about your thoughts, you can choose to think good thoughts and feel good, or you can choose to think bad thoughts and feel lousy. Through cognitive, or thought, therapy, you can learn how to change your thoughts and change the way you feel. One way to learn how to change your thoughts is to notice them when they are negative and talk back to them. If you think a negative thought without challenging it, your mind believes it and your body reacts to it.

ANTs and ANTeaters*

Children have trouble understanding the principle of directed thoughts (as do many adults). As a child psychiatrist, Dr. Amen developed an analogy to help children understand and correct negative thoughts. He called them "automatic negative thoughts," or ANTs, named after the little red or black insects that can invade the kitchen. Having bad thoughts is like having an ANT invasion in your head. When you feel sad, blue, anxious, or mad, an ANT invasion is often fueling the bad feelings. You need a strong, internal ANTeater to get rid of the ANTs and the bad feelings that follow. Unless you crush the ANTs, they will ruin your mood, your sense of internal calm, your relationships, and your self-esteem and personal power. One way to crush these ANTs is to write them down and talk back to them. By doing so, you take away their power. You do not have to accept every thought that goes through your mind.

There are nine different ANT species, or ways that your thoughts can lie to you to make situations out to be worse than they really are. Some of these ANTs are designated as red because they are particularly harmful to you. ANTeating strategies are discussed beginning on page 193.

Readers of Dr. Amen's previous work will be familiar with ANT therapy. We feel it is an essential strategy for coping with anxiety and depression.

ANT #1: "Always Thinking"

These ANTs occur when you overgeneralize a situation and think something that happened once will "always" repeat itself. For example, if your wife snaps at you, you may think, "She's always irritable," even though she may only have snapped once. The thought "She's always irritable" is so negative that it makes you feel sad and upset. It activates your limbic system. Whenever you think in absolutes such as "always," "never," "no one," "everyone," "every time," or "everything," you are engaging in negative thinking that seems to make a temporary situation a permanent reality. Here are some examples of "always" thinking:

"He's *always* angry."

"*No one* is concerned about my ideas."

"He *never* listens to me."

"*Everyone* takes advantage of me."

"You turn away *every time* I touch you."

"My kids *always* disrespect me."

"Always thinking" ANTs are very common. Beware when they creep into your thinking (and conversations) as they can have a very negative effect on your mood, attitude, and relationships.

ANT #2 (red ANT): "Focusing on the Negative"

These ANTs occur when you focus only on what's going wrong in a situation and ignore everything that could be construed as positive. This ANT can take a positive experience, relationship, or work interaction and taint it with negativity. For example, you feel a deep desire to help a neighbor in need and you have the means and knowledge to help, but as you prepare to step in, you remember a time when the neighbor disappointed you. Even though you have had many positive encounters with your neighbor, you become focused on the negative event. The negativity causes you to pause in your effort to help, and then you get distracted by other things and forget to help. Another example: You have a wonderful date with someone you just met. Everything goes well—you are attracted to her spirit, her mind, her values, and her looks, except she was ten minutes late for the date. If you choose to focus on her being late, you can ruin a potentially wonderful relationship. Or say you go to a new church or synagogue. It is a very fulfilling experience, except someone makes too much noise and distracts you during part of the service. If you focus on the disruption, you might not go back and you may lose out on a wonderful opportunity for fellowship.

Your deep limbic system can learn a powerful lesson from the Disney movie *Pollyanna*. In the movie, Pollyanna goes to live with her aunt after the death of her missionary parents. Although an orphan, Pollyanna is able to help many "negative people" with her positive attitude when she introduces them to the "glad game" her father taught her. Pollyanna first played the glad game when her parents requested a doll for her from their missionary sponsors and mistakenly received crutches instead. Rather than be upset at not having a doll, Pollyanna's father taught her she could be glad because they didn't need crutches. This very simple game changes the attitudes and lives of many people in the movie. Pollyanna has a particular effect on the unhappy "hell and damnation" minister. Pollyanna tells him that her father said there were 800 "glad passages" in the Bible and that if God mentioned being glad that many times, it must be because He wants us to think that way.

Focusing on the negative in situations will make you feel bad. Playing the glad game, or looking for the positive, will help you feel better.

ANT #3 (red ANT): "Fortune Telling"

These ANTs occur when you predict that bad or negative things will happen. Fortune-telling ANTs underlie most anxiety disorders, especially with people who have panic attacks. Predicting the worst in a situation causes an immediate rise in heart and breathing rates. Having these thoughts can make you feel tense. These fortune-telling ANTs are designated "red" because, when you predict that bad things will happen, you may find yourself experiencing them. If, for example, you are driving to work and you predict that you'll have a bad day, the first bad thing that happens will reinforce your belief and the rest of the day will go downhill. While it's important to be prepared for potential negative events or outcomes, overfocusing on them will damage your peace of mind and ultimately ruin your health.

> *Dr. Amen: I have struggled with fortune-telling ANTs throughout my life. I know how they can cause a pervasive sense of fear and anxiety. When I first*

started my brain imaging research, I decided to study the brain patterns of my own family, including my mother, my aunt, my wife, my three children, and myself. I wanted to see if the patterns I was seeing correlated with the people with whom I had the most intimate knowledge. I quickly learned that getting my own brain scanned was not an easy experience. Even with all that I have intellectually accomplished in my life, I was still very anxious about the procedure. What if something was wrong with my brain? What if nothing was there at all? I never felt more naked than after my scan, when my own brain activity was projected onto a computer screen in front of my colleagues. At that moment, I would rather have been without clothes than without the covering of my skull. I was relieved to see very good activity in nearly all of my brain. I saw an area of overactivity in the right side of my basal ganglia, however, that stood out like a red Christmas tree light bulb. The part of the brain that often sets off anxiety was working too hard. This discovery made sense to me. Although I do not have a clinical disorder, such as Panic Disorder, I have struggled my whole life with minor issues of anxiety. I used to bite my nails and sometimes still do when I feel anxious. I used to find it very difficult to ask for payment from patients after therapy sessions. I also had a terrible time speaking in front of large groups (which now I love to do). My first appearance on television was terrible. My hands sweated so much that I unknowingly rubbed them on my pants throughout the interview. Right before my second television interview, I nearly had a panic attack. While I was sitting in the greenroom waiting to go on the air, my mind became flooded with fortune-telling ANTs, and I began to predict disaster. I thought I would make a fool of myself, forget my own name, say something stupid, stutter or stumble over my words, and basically make an idiot of myself in front of 2 million people. Thankfully, I recognized what was happening to me and chuckled to myself: "I treat people who have this problem. Breathe with your belly and kill the ANTs."

ANT #4 (red ANT): "Mind Reading"

Mind-reading ANTs occur when you think you know what others are thinking even when they haven't told you. Mind reading is a common cause of trouble between people. It frequently happens in intimate relationships because one partner assumes he can read the other's mind—but you can never know what others are thinking. You know you are mind reading when you have thoughts such as, "He doesn't like me." "They were talking about me." "They think I will never amount to much." I tell people that a negative look from someone else may be nothing more than his being constipated! You just don't know. When there are things you don't understand, ask for clarification and stay away from mind-reading ANTs. They are very infectious and cause trouble between people.

ANT #5: "Thinking with Your Feelings"

These ANTs occur when you believe your negative feelings without ever questioning them. Feelings are very complex and are often based on powerful memories from the past. Feelings sometimes lie but many people believe their feelings even though they have no evidence to back them up. "Thinking with your feelings" thoughts usually start with the words "I feel." For example, "I feel like you don't love me." "I feel stupid." "I feel like a failure." "I feel nobody will ever trust me." Whenever you have a strong negative feeling, check it out. Look for the evidence behind the feeling. Do you have real reasons to feel that way? Or are your feelings based on events or things from the past?

ANT #6: "Guilt Beatings"

Guilt is generally not a helpful emotion, especially for your deep limbic system. In fact, guilt often causes you to do things that you don't want to do. Guilt beatings happen when you think with words like "should," "must," "ought," or "have to." Here are some examples: "I *ought* to spend more time at home." "I *must* spend more time with my kids." "I *should* have sex more often." "I *have* to organize my office." Guilt-inducing behaviors are common in many religious institutions. "Live your life this way or else bad things will happen to you" is a frequent message. Of course there are things that you should not do. Moral teaching is very important. Yet when the goal of teaching is to produce guilt, it is often counterproductive. Unfortunately, guilt often backfires. Because of human nature, whenever we think that we "must" do something, no matter what it is, we don't want to do it. It is better to replace "guilt beatings" with phrases such as "I want to do this . . ." "It fits with my goals to do that . . ." "It would be helpful to do this . . ." In the examples above, it would be helpful to change those phrases to "I want to spend more time at home." "It's in our best interest for my kids and me to spend more time together." "I want to please my spouse by making wonderful love with him [or her] because he [or she] is important to me." "It's in my best interest to organize my office." Get rid of the unnecessary emotional turbulence that holds you back from achieving the goals you want.

ANT #7: "Labeling"

Whenever you attach a negative label to yourself or to someone else, you prevent yourself from taking a clear look at the situation. Some examples of negative labels that people use are "jerk," "frigid," "arrogant," and "irresponsible." Negative labels are very harmful because whenever you call yourself or someone else a jerk or arrogant, you lump that person in your mind with all the "jerks" or "arrogant people" that you've ever known and you become unable to deal with them in a reasonable way. Stay away from negative labels.

ANT #8: "Personalization"

Personalization occurs when innocuous events are taken personally—"My boss didn't talk to me this morning. She must be mad at me"—or, one feels he or she is the cause of all the bad things that happen—"My son got into a car accident. I should have spent more time teaching him to drive. It must be my fault." There are many other possible reasons for behavior besides the negative interpretations of an abnormal limbic system. For example, your boss may not have talked to you because she was preoccupied or upset, or she was in a hurry. You never fully know why people do what they do. Try not to personalize their behavior.

ANT #9 (the most poisonous red ANT): "Blame"

Blame is very harmful. When you blame something or someone else for the problems in your life, you become a victim of circumstances and you cannot do anything to change your situation. Many relationships are ruined by people who blame their partners when things go wrong. They take little responsibility for or won't admit to their problems. When something goes wrong at home or at work, they try to find someone to blame. Typically, you'll hear statements from them such as:

"It wasn't my fault that . . ."

"That wouldn't have happened if you had . . ."

"How was I supposed to know . . ."

"It's your fault that . . ."

The bottom-line statement goes something like this: "If only you had done something differently, I wouldn't be in the predicament I'm in. It's your fault, and I'm not responsible."

Whenever you blame someone else for the problems in your life, you become powerless to change anything. The "blame game" hurts your personal sense of power. Stay away from blaming thoughts and take personal responsibility for your problems.

In order to keep your brain functioning at a high level, it is important to have good emotional and thought management. Whenever you notice an ANT entering your mind, train yourself to recognize it and write it down. When

---

Killing the ANTs

This exercise is for whenever you need to be in control of your mind. It is for times when you feel anxious, nervous, depressed, or frazzled. It is for times when you need to be your best.

EVENT: Describe the event that is associated with your thoughts and feelings.

_____

_____

_____

_____

ANT	Species	Kill the ANT
(write out the automatic negative thoughts)	(identify the type of irrational thought)	(talk back to the irrational thoughts)
_____	_____	_____
_____	_____	_____
_____	_____	_____
_____	_____	_____
_____	_____	_____
_____	_____	_____
_____	_____	_____

Here are some examples of ways to kill these ANTs:

ANT	Species	Kill the ANT
You never listen to me.	Always Thinking	I get frustrated when you don't listen to me, but I know you have listened to me and will again.
The minister doesn't like me.	Mind Reading	I don't know that. Maybe he's just having a bad day. Ministers are people, too.
I'll stutter if I do the reading at church.	Fortune Telling	I don't know that. Odds are I will do fine.
I'm unlovable.	Labeling	Sometimes I do things that push others away, but I can find love and be in a loving relationship.
It's your fault we have these problems.	Blame	I need to look at my part of the problems and look for ways I can make the situation better.

you write down automatic negative thoughts (ANTs) and talk back to them, you begin to take away their power and gain control over your moods.

Your thoughts matter. They can either help or hurt your deep limbic system. Left unchecked, ANTs will cause an infection in your whole body system. Whenever you notice ANTs, you need to crush them or they'll affect your relationships, your work, and your life. If you can catch them at the moment they occur and correct them, you take away their power over you. When a negative thought goes unchallenged, your mind believes it and your body reacts to it.

ANTs have an illogical logic. By bringing them into the open and examining them on a conscious level, you can see for yourself how little sense it makes to think these kinds of things. You take back control of your own life instead of leaving your fate to hyperactive limbic–conditioned negative thought patterns.

Sometimes people have trouble talking back to these grossly unpleasant thoughts because they feel that such obvious age-old "truisms" simply must be real. They think that if they don't continue to believe these thoughts they are lying to themselves. Once again, remember that to know what is true and what is not, you have to be conscious of the thoughts. Most negative thinking is automatic and goes unnoticed. You're not really choosing how to respond to your situation, it's being chosen for you, by bad brain habits. To find out what is really true and what is not, you need to question. Don't believe everything you hear—even in your own mind!

We often ask our patients about their ANT population. Is it high? Low? Dwindling? Increasing? Keep control over the ANTs in order to maintain a healthy deep limbic environment.

CHAPTER 11

The Healing Power
of Relationships

Relationships are critical to human health. Having a healthy brain helps you make and maintain connections with others. In his wonderful book *Love and Survival,* cardiologist Dean Ornish details the many benefits from having close relationships. Dr. Ornish cites numerous studies indicating that those who feel close, connected, loved, and supported have a lower incidence of depression, anxiety, suicide, heart disease, infections, hypertension, and cancer. Love enhances brain function, and a healthy brain enhances our ability to love and be connected to others.

One of the most striking findings of Dr. Amen's seven years as a military psychiatrist was that, according to military statistics, the incidence of suicides and suicide attempts among military service personnel and their dependents peaks in the months of January and July; in a civilian population, suicide is highest in April. What was responsible for the discrepancy in the two populations? January and July are the months of military moves, and when people move they become disconnected from their social support network and are at greater risk for depression and suicide. Dr. Amen frequently treated military wives who became depressed for six months after a move. Their depression seemed to lift after they developed a new social network— friends, church, social groups. The women who did not become depressed were much more skilled at getting involved and developing social support right away. Suicide in a civilian population may peak in April because people who experienced winter depressions may be coming out of them with increased energy to act on their bad thoughts. It could also be because April is tax time.

Having strong social support networks can also delay the brain's aging process. Maintaining relationships and participating in social activities have been associated with improved memory and intelligence in the elderly. Not at all coincidentally, social isolation is considered a risk factor for cognitive decline. In a study reported in 1999 in the *Annals of Internal Medicine,* 2,812 community-dwelling persons sixty-five years or older were followed for up to twelve years. Social isolation at the beginning of the study, as measured by the absence of such things as a spouse, contact with friends or relatives, and participation in group activities, was significantly associated with subsequent worsening of cognitive impairment as measured by a questionnaire. Social isolation was also associated with increased illness and earlier death.

Social bonding is one of the key principles behind the success of support groups such as Alcoholics Anonymous. For years, clinicians have known that one of the best ways to help people with serious problems such as alcoholism is to get them to connect with others who have the same problem. By seeing how others have learned from their experiences and coped with tough times in positive ways, alcoholics can find the way out of their own plight. While gaining information about the disease is helpful, forming new relationships and connections with others may be the critical link in the chain of recovery.

Enhancing emotional bonds between people enhances brain function. In one large study in which patients were treated for major depression, the National Institutes of Health compared three approaches: antidepressant medication, cognitive therapy (similar to ANT therapy discussed earlier), and interpersonal psychotherapy (enhancing relationship skills). Researchers were surprised to find that each of the treatments was equally effective in treating depression. (Many people in the medical community think that the benefits of medication far outweigh the benefits of therapy.) Not surprising was the fact that combining all three treatments had an even more powerful effect. Not only were pharmaceuticals and professional therapists helpful, but patients played a significant role in helping each other. How you get along with other people can either help or hurt your limbic system! Our day-to-day interactions with others enhance or hurt how the brain works. Being more connected to the people in your life helps to heal the brain. Love is as powerful as drugs and usually a lot more fun.

The improvements patients with depression obtain from interpersonal psychotherapy (IPT) appear to go all the way to the brain, according to research reported by Dr. Stephen D. Martin of the University of Durham in Sunderland, England. Brain SPECT studies show that the function of brain structures critical to mood regulation can return to normal after a short course of IPT. "We're starting to see some fascinating consistency in the data," Dr. Martin said at the annual meeting of the American Psychiatric Association in 1999. Researchers at the university's Cherry Knowle Hospital performed SPECT studies on twenty-seven adult patients with major depression. The investigators then randomly assigned fourteen of the patients to receive the antidepressant venlafaxine, while thirteen other patients began weekly one-hour IPT sessions. After six weeks of treatment, depression scores improved significantly in both groups. A second round of SPECT studies after treatment in both groups also showed significant improvement, especially in the areas of the deep limbic system and anterior cingulate gyrus, indicating that patients were less depressed and less overfocused on bad feelings. The imaging findings, according to Dr. Martin, support the notion that brain changes contribute significantly to both the development and the resolution of major depression. "We may be looking at a pattern of holistic etiology in which both targeted psychotherapy and medication can influence neurophysiology," he said.

In another groundbreaking effort to make a quantitative comparison of therapies for depression, Arthur L. Brody, M.D., assistant professor of psychiatry at the University of California, Los Angeles' (UCLA) Neuropsychiatric Institute, used positron emission tomography (PET) scans to observe brain changes in patients receiving IPT as compared to patients receiving psychopharmacological therapy. Funded by an award from the National Association for Research on Schizophrenia and Depression (NARSAD), Brody, who is also director of UCLA's Interpersonal Psychotherapy Clinic, wrote that in functional imaging studies, the brain regions most commonly found to have abnormalities in major depression are the prefrontal cortex, anterior cingulate gyrus, temporal cortex, and basal ganglia. Therefore, he and his colleagues sought to determine metabolic changes in these regions in subjects with major depression from pre- to posttreatment with either paroxetine (Paxil) or IPT. In a published preliminary study in which his group used PET scans to examine changes in sixteen depressed subjects treated with paroxetine, he reported at a national scientific meeting, "What we did there is compare responders to treatment to nonresponders. And what we found is that responders to treatment had decreases in activity in the prefrontal cortex and the orbital frontal cortex, the part of the cortex right above the eyes. That's a region that has strong input from the serotonin system, so that might explain why that region had a decrease in activity when subjects were treated with a serotonin reuptake inhibitor. Nonresponders did not have these decreases in activity." Brody explained that the goal of IPT is to improve depressive symptoms through strengthening the patient's interpersonal relationships. "The focus is on current stressors in a person's life and practical ways to improve relationships to alleviate those stressors and strengthen existing relationships," he said. "It's a very direct therapy where we use behavior change techniques and actually suggest alternatives for patients to do in their current relationships. The therapist in this therapy is a patient advocate, not neutral . . . and active, not passive. It's a very interactive type of psychotherapy."

In the IPT study, twenty-four study subjects with major depression were allowed to choose either IPT or medication therapy. This resulted in fourteen subjects in the psychotherapy group and ten in the paroxetine group. Also included were sixteen normal controls who received no psychotherapy or medication. All subjects were scanned twice, about twelve weeks apart. Pre- and postmeasures of mood were evaluated. "This was a slightly sicker group overall than in our previous study of depression, in that the people in the IPT group had an average of 3.5 previous treatments for depression, and the paroxetine group had 2.1 previous episodes," Brody noted. "The IPT group also started out with a slightly higher depression rating than the paroxetine group." Results for the paroxetine-treated subjects showed a 62 percent drop in their depression scores, whereas, for the psychotherapy subjects, there was only about a 40 percent drop in scores. Brody said that, as in the previous study, PET scans of the paroxetine patients showed a decrease in activity in the prefrontal cortex. "Finding this decrease in both of our studies of patients treated with Paxil makes this a much stronger finding," he said. "These were two different groups of subjects and done on two different scanners with slightly different methods, and we found the same thing. Other groups have had similar findings as well." In the IPT group, PET scans showed a highly significant increase in activity in the inferior frontal gyrus and anterior insula for all subjects. Normal controls had no significant change on their PET scans other than normal changes seen with repeated scans. "This is an area that's been associated with language," Brody said of the inferior frontal gyrus and anterior insula region. "It's also been associated with movement and emotion. So one of our hypotheses is that maybe after the talk therapy they received, they were thinking about talking more, or more talkative in general." Asked about long-term implications of medication versus psychotherapy, Brody said,

"What actually tends to happen is that people who get treated with IPT . . . tend to maintain better social functioning later on. But in terms of who does better in the long run, medication and psychotherapy both have strengths and weaknesses. Neither therapy has definitively been proven superior to the other, but some studies have shown superior efficacy for medication as perhaps being a little more effective than psychotherapy (in more severely depressed individuals). But the people who get the psychotherapy tend to have better social functioning one, two, or three years out of the psychotherapy."

People Are Contagious

Who you spend time with matters. When you are with positive, supportive, and loving people, you feel happier and more content, and you live longer. This is not only intuitively true but research has demonstrated it again and again. For example, in a study at Case Western Reserve in Cleveland, Ohio, 10,000 men were asked, "Does your wife show you her love?" The detailed health histories of the men followed over ten years who answered yes showed fewer ulcers, less chest pain, and longer lives than those who answered no.

When you spend time with negative or hostile people, you tend to feel tense, anxious, upset, sick, and less intellectually on the ball. Being around people who make you feel stress causes your body to secrete excessive amounts of adrenaline, which makes you feel anxious and tense and puts you on your guard. Increases in the stress hormone cortisol can disrupt neurons in the hippocampus, one of the main memory centers in the brain. Through the years people have told us that living with a person who suffered from Schizophrenia, Bipolar Disorder, Depression, Panic Disorder, Attention Deficit Disorder, or Borderline Personality Disorder has had a negative impact on their physical and emotional health. The chronic stress for family members associated with these illnesses when they are untreated or undertreated can be devastating. Mothers of untreated ADD children, for example, have a higher incidence of depression themselves and often complain that they are physically sick more often and cognitively less sharp than before they had the child.

In our experience, a hallmark of unhappy people is that they have a tendency to surround themselves with negative people—with people who do not believe in them or their abilities, people who put them down, discourage them from their goals, and treat them as though they will never amount to anything. Surrounded by these types of people, you eventually get a clear message that you are no good.

Are you surrounded by people who believe in you and give you positive messages? People who encourage you to feel good about yourself? Or do you spend time with people who are constantly putting you down and downplaying your ideas? Who are the five people you spend the most time with? Are they positive or negative? The reasons people surround themselves with negativity are easy to understand. People who grow up in negative environments often grow up to be negative. It is what they are used to and, in a strange sort of way, it is what they are comfortable with, what their brain knows. A Choctaw medicine man once told us, "People do not seek happiness, they seek familiarity." If an insecure parent continually belittles his child to make himself feel better, the child grows up believing that he is no good and that he is not worthy of being around people who make him feel good. When the trauma of divorce or death happens in a family, a young child often erroneously believes he is at fault and carries around tremendous guilt for a long time. Some children who witnessed parents struggle through a difficult marriage get the message programmed in their brains that relationships are inherently problematic, and they, too, get caught in incompatible relationships.

Adults as well as children can be beaten down after years of living through a difficult marriage or being in an abusive job situation. Many people will stay in a job they hate, for example, because their boss leads them to believe that no one else would hire them and that they are lucky to have the job. Just as in an abusive marriage, in an abusive job situation employees have their self-esteem beaten down to the point that they no longer believe they can go beyond their abusive environment.

Past relationships have a real impact on present ones. If your past relationships were filled with negativity, chances are your present and future relationships will be the same unless you make a conscious effort to overcome the past.

Enhancing Social Support and Connections

It takes effort to overcome difficult foundational relationships, but it is possible. Changing the people you spend time with may be an important step in changing your mood or anxiety level. A positive environment is growth-enhancing; a negative one chokes and suffocates growth.

Inventory Your Interactions

In order to change your interactions with those around you, you must first get an idea of who you spend the most time with and what those relationships are like. List the five people with whom you spend the most time. Then answer the following questions about each relationship:

How much time do you spend with each of the people on your list?

In what contexts or situations do you come together?

Do you look forward to being with that person?

How do you feel prior to seeing him?

How does she treat you when you're with her?

Is he critical or supportive?

Does she make overtly hostile remarks, or does she abuse you in a more subtle way?

How do you treat him?

How do you feel when you're with her?

Are you able to hear what she has to say without being defensive?

How do you feel when you're away from him?

After you answer these questions, rate each of the relationships on a 1-to-10 scale, with 1 being a very negative relationship, and 10 being an uplifting and supportive relationship. Use this information to evaluate your relationships to see which ones you like and which you need to work on.

Change the Negative Interactions

We all teach others how to interact with and respond to us. If, by our actions, we teach them that they must respect us or we'll have nothing to do with them, they either treat us with respect or we cut them from our lives. If we teach them that we'll accept their negative comments or verbal or physical abuse, they may continue to abuse us. Be clear and consistent about the bottom line. Quite often, low self-esteem gets in the way of good boundary setting, and some of us accept the abuse because somehow we think we deserve it. Abuse is never deserved or appropriate.

Once relational patterns are established, they can be changed. Follow these six steps to changing your negative interactions with others:

1. Recognize and be clear about what, specifically, each of you do to contribute to the negative interaction.

2. Take responsibility for what you do to add to the negative situation— and change it.

3. Tell people they are important to you (if they weren't, you wouldn't be bothering with them), and that some of the things they do cause you to feel hurt or put down. Be specific: "When you cut me down in front of other people, it really hurts my feelings."

4. Ask them to change. First, tell them how upset their behavior makes you feel, and then ask them to change it. (Often, this is all it takes.)

5. If asking doesn't change the behavior, make it uncomfortable for them to treat you that way, i.e., "If you do that again, I'll let you know—I won't allow you to treat me like that in front of others!" Make it clear which behaviors you'll accept and which you won't. Be ready to back up words with action.

6. If that still doesn't work, raise the stakes. In order for change to take place, the person must feel uncomfortable, sometimes very uncom- fortable. Often this may mean threatening to terminate the relation- ship unless a person is willing to get help. Negative relationships take more out of you physically and emotionally than they are usually worth.

Before you get out of negative relationships, you need more informa- tion: Can you change your interactions? Can the other person change his? If others are teachable, you need to teach them how to treat you. Whether or not you recognize it, you've been doing that all along. If you find your- self unable to teach others to treat you with respect, odds are it's because you believe you don't deserve respect. If that's the case, you may need profes- sional assistance to help you develop your self-worth.

Decrease the Time You Spend with Those Who Put You Down

If the negative people in your environment are unwilling or unable to change, decrease the amount of time you spend with them. Remember, if your environment is negative, so are you. Obviously, you may not be able to totally eliminate your interactions with some of these people, such as parents or close relatives. But you don't have to spend as much time with them. The time is better spent with those who uplift or encourage you.

Here are some actions to take:

- Call them only half as much, or wait for them to call you.

- If they start in on you, find a way to get off the phone.

- Spend your coffee breaks with new people.

- If you need to communicate with them, write them a letter.

- Keep a schedule of things to do so that when they ask you out, you don't say yes out of boredom.

At the same time, you need to establish new, positive relationships. When you meet someone who adds good things to your life, take care of the relationship. Call, be kind, be interested. Following are some ideas on ways to meet new, more positive people:

- Go to five different congregations in five weeks—see in which one the people make you feel most comfortable.

- Join a support group.

- Go to lunch with someone new, someone you may never have thought you'd like to have lunch with—expand your horizons.

- Take a fun class at your local community college or through an adult education program, even if you already have a degree.

- Start a new hobby, one that includes other people—sailing, hiking, table tennis, square dancing, volleyball or any team sport, photography, or volunteering for a local service agency. The possibilities are endless.

Keys to Effective Relationships

Here are eleven relational principles to help maintain social connections and keep deep limbic systems healthy:

1. *Take responsibility for keeping your relationships strong.* Don't be the one who blames your partner or your friends for the problems in the relationship. Take responsibility for the relationship and look for what you can do to improve it. You'll feel empowered, and the relationship is likely to improve almost immediately. Taking responsibility does not mean blaming yourself for all of the problems, but it also means not blaming others for all of the problems, either. It starts with the question "What can I do today to make our relationship better?" Blaming others for relationship problems is easy, almost natural, but very destructive.

2. *Never take the relationship for granted.* In order for relationships to be special they need constant nurturing. Relationships suffer when they are low on the priority list of time and attention. Take time every day to let the people in your lives know you love them. You need love like you need air and nutrition. Focus energy on your relationships to help them stay satisfying.

3. *Protect your relationship.* A surefire way to doom a relationship is to discount, belittle, or degrade the other person. Protect your relationships by building up the other person. Notice what you like about the people in your life more than what you do not like. You shape the behavior of others by how you treat them.

4. *Assume the best.* Whenever there is a question of motivation or intention, assume the best about the other person. Motivation is complex and often hard to understand. Assuming the worst about someone most often causes isolation, cynicism, and loneliness. Even if you occasionally err in your judgment, overall you will have much more support in your life to deal with the disappointments. Some people tell us that they are pessimistic and distrusting, and that way they are never disappointed. While there may be less chance of being disappointed with this approach, they will likely die sooner than those who have a more positive attitude toward others.

5. *Keep relationships fresh.* When relationships become stale or boring, they become vulnerable to erosion. Stay away from "the same old

thing" by looking for new and different ways to add life to your relationships. The brain accommodates routine. When you do the same thing over and over, the brain actually uses less energy (it already knows how to do routine) and becomes sluggish or looks for more interesting pursuits. To keep relationships and the brain young and healthy, come up with new and different ways of doing things with those you love.

6. *Notice the good.* It's very easy to notice what you do not like about a relationship. That's almost our nature. It takes real effort to notice what you like. When you spend more time noticing the positive aspects of the relationship, you're more likely to see an increase in positive behavior.

7. *Communicate clearly.* Most fights people have stem from some form of miscommunication. Take time to really listen and understand what other people say to you. Don't react to what you think someone means; ask them what they mean and then formulate a response.

8. *Maintain and protect trust.* So many relationships fall apart after there has been a major violation of trust, such as an affair or other form of dishonesty. Often hurts in the present, even minor ones, remind us of major traumas in the past and we blow them way out of proportion. Once trust has been violated, try to understand why it happened, since it is usually a symptom of ongoing relationship issues and rarely the primary problem.

9. *Deal with difficult issues.* Whenever you give in to another person to avoid a fight, you give away a little of your power. If you do this over time, you give away a lot of power and begin to resent the relationship. Avoiding conflict in the short run often has devastating long-term effects. In a firm but kind way stick up for what you know is right. It will help keep the relationship balanced. This means sticking with an exchange until you have been able to convince your partner to "come over to your side," until your partner has persuaded you that they have the better idea, or until the two of you come up with a compromise plan that is satisfactory to both of you.

10. *Time.* In our busy lives, time is often the first thing to suffer in our important relationships. Relationships require real time in order to

function. Many couples today find themselves in the situation where both partners are working and parenting children, and they gradually grow apart because they have no time together. When they do get time together, they often realize how much they really like each other. Make your special relationships a "time investment" and it will pay dividends for years to come.

11. *Touch is necessary for humans.* The limbic brain is involved not only in emotional bonding, but in physical bonding as well. Physical connection is also a critical element in the parent-infant bonding process and the developing brain. The caressing, kissing, sweet words, and eye contact from parents give a baby the pleasure, love, trust, and security it needs to develop healthy deep limbic pathways. Without love and affection, a baby does not develop appropriate deep limbic connectedness and thus never learns to trust or connect. He feels lonely and insecure and grows irritable and unresponsive. Touch is critical to life itself. In a barbaric thirteenth-century experiment, the German emperor Frederick II wanted to know what language and words children would speak if they were raised without hearing any words at all. He took a number of infants from their homes and placed them with people who fed them but who had strict instructions not to touch, cuddle, or talk to them. The babies never spoke a word. They all died before they could speak. Even though the language experiment was a failure, it is an important discovery. Touch is essential to life. Salimbene, historian of the time, wrote of the experiment in 1248: "They could not live without petting." This powerful finding has been rediscovered over and over, most recently in the early 1990s in Romania, where thousands of orphaned, "warehoused" infants went without touch for up to years at a time. Many of these children developed serious behavioral problems such as social aloofness, aggressive behavior, and learning problems. We have performed a number of SPECT studies on such children and have seen firsthand that the absence of human connection causes decreased activity in all areas of the brain.

Social connections are necessary for a healthy brain, and a healthy brain makes positive social connections more likely. Connectedness is the essence of our humanity. Strive to be closer to someone today and make it a top priority in your life.

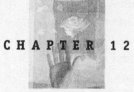

CHAPTER 12

Gaining Self-Control: Breathing and Biofeedback Strategies

Eight-year-old Brenna suffered from excessive shyness and severe anxiety. She hid behind her mother when introduced to strangers, rarely spoke during school classes, ate lunch by herself, and often complained of stomachaches and headaches. Her father had had similar problems when he was a child and had been diagnosed with Generalized Anxiety Disorder as an adult. After a thorough evaluation at our clinic, Brenna was diagnosed with Type 1, Pure Anxiety. As part of her treatment we hooked her up to our computerized biofeedback equipment. We measured her hand temperature, heart rate, breathing patterns, hand sweat gland activity, and muscle tension. All of these physiological systems were running on overload. It was as if she were living in a constant state of fear, living in a fight-or-flight "adrenalized" state. Her hands were cold, her heart beat faster than her peers', her breathing was rapid and shallow, and her muscles were tense. Brenna spent most of her days overwhelmed by anxiety. Using playful computer games in which she learned to change her body's own physiology, we taught her how to warm her hands, lower her heart rate, slow and deepen her breathing, relax her muscles, and dry her hands. During three months of biofeedback training, Brenna showed signs of progressive relaxation. Her physical symptoms of stress (headaches and stomachaches) lessened, she was able to talk in class and became more social, and she was more comfortable in her own skin.

Biofeedback is based on a very simple concept. If you get feedback on a physiological process in the body, such as breathing, hand temperature, sweat gland activity, heart rate, muscle tension, or brainwave patterns, you can learn to control it over time. Biofeedback has been compared to looking in a mirror after waking in the morning. Once you look in the mirror, you can adjust your appearance to be more presentable. The mirror gives you feedback on how you look, and you use the feedback to make helpful adjustments. Biofeedback and self-regulation have been part of psychotherapy treatment regimens since the late 1960s. With the advent of computer technology in the late 1980s, biofeedback equipment has become an amazingly helpful technology in adjusting the body's physiological processes. Unfortunately, the technology is underutilized. The concept of biofeedback has been pivotal in Dr. Amen's thought process of various anxiety and depressive disorders.

Dr. Amen: After my psychiatric training programs at Walter Reed Army Medical Center in Washington, D.C., and Tripler Army Medical Center in Honolulu, Hawaii, I was stationed at Fort Irwin, forty miles north of Barstow, in California's Mojave Desert. Halfway between Los Angeles and Las Vegas, Fort Irwin was also known as the National Training Center where American soldiers were taught to fight the Russians (and later the Iraqis) in the desert. At the time, I was the only psychiatrist for 4,000 soldiers and an equal number of family members. It was an isolated assignment for all of us. At Fort Irwin, there were problems with domestic violence, drug abuse (especially amphetamine abuse), depression, and ailments resulting from the stress of living in the middle of nowhere. I dealt with many people who suffered from headaches, anxiety attacks, insomnia, and excessive muscle tension.

Shortly after arriving at Fort Irwin, I went through the cabinets in the community mental health clinic to see what instruments and psychological tests my predecessors had left behind. To my delight, there was an old Autogen biofeedback apparatus that measured hand temperature. While I had had only one lecture on biofeedback during my psychiatric training, the concept of self-regulation fascinated me. The problem with biofeedback was that the training was boring. The needles and dials on the machines were not interesting to patients. Nonetheless, we used the old machine with patients who had migraine headaches. I taught them how to warm their hands using only their imagination, which helps with migraines because it increases the body's relaxation response, which counteracts the stress often associated with headaches. It was fascinating to see how patients could actually increase their hand temperature, sometimes by as much as 15 to 20 degrees. Hand-temperature training was helpful for many patients. It allowed them to participate in their own healing process, rather than relying on medication to take away the pain.

Six months after coming to Fort Irwin, I wrote to Colonel Knowles, our hospital commander, requesting permission to buy the mental health clinic $30,000 worth of the latest computerized biofeedback equipment, including ten days of training for me in San Francisco. He laughed at my request. He said that the army didn't have that kind of money, and that when my assignment at Fort Irwin was over the equipment would just end up in a closet somewhere, much like the equipment I had found. I dropped the idea, but continued using the old temperature trainer. Nearly a year later I was surprised to have my request authorized. In the army, if a unit does not spend its entire annual budget, they lose the unspent portion the next year. The unit's unspent budget went for new equipment, and ten days' training in San Francisco!

The biofeedback training course at the Applied Psychophysiological Institute (API) in San Francisco changed my life. It was the most stimulating and intense learning experience I had had as a physician. The ten-hour days went by in a flash. The new computerized biofeedback equipment was patient-friendly, interesting, and easy to learn. I learned how to help people relax their muscles, warm their hands (much faster than with the old equipment), calm sweat gland activity, lower blood pressure, slow their own heart rates, and breathe in ways that promoted relaxation.

The lectures on brainwave biofeedback were the most amazing. I was taught that people can actually learn how to change their own brainwave patterns. What an exciting concept it was to be able to change your own mental state. I also learned about Dr. Joel Lubar's research at the University of Tennessee on brainwave underactivity in children with ADD and about other researchers and doctors who used brainwave biofeedback for depression, anxiety, and substance abuse.

When I returned to Fort Irwin, I tried everything I had learned. I did biofeedback on almost all the patients who came to see me. I loved it. My patients loved it. I also spent time each day doing it myself. I became a master at breathing with my diaphragm. I could slow my heart rate. And I could even warm my hands whenever I felt stressed. I also started to evaluate children with ADD by using EEG measures. Many of them demonstrated the same patterns that Dr. Lubar had written about, and many of them benefited from biofeedback training.

When my commitment to the U.S. Army ended, I started a private practice in Fairfield, California. I bought my own biofeedback equipment and continued using it in clinical practice. Also, when I became the medical director of the dual diagnosis unit (where patients had both substance abuse and psychiatric problems) at a local psychiatric hospital, I instituted the use of biofeedback throughout the hospital.

I continue to use biofeedback to this day.

Biofeedback has its roots in the medical literature on stress and the fight-or-flight response. Scientists have known for many decades that the brain has a system to calm the body (the parasympathetic system) and a system to activate the body or get it ready to deal with a specific stress or fear (the sympathetic nervous system). The sympathetic system, when stimulated, is responsible for the fight-or-flight response, a primitive state that gets us ready to fight or flee when we are threatened or scared. This "hard-wired response" happens with overt physical threats (such as being approached by a vicious dog) and also with more covert, internal, emotional threats (such as a self-esteem injury or worry about the future). The heart beats faster, muscles tense, hands sweat to cool the body, breathing rate and blood pressure increase, the hands and feet become cooler to shunt blood from the extremities to the big muscles (to fight or run away), and the pupils dilate (to see better). This response to stress is powerful and immediate. Psychological trauma also inflames the emotional centers of the brain and resets our bodies to a higher, more stressed level, causing a constant outflow of the fight-or-flight response.

Using biofeedback equipment, we have performed many psychophysiological stress tests. It is a fascinating process to watch. We monitor a person's heart rate, breathing rate, hand temperature, hand sweat gland activity, and muscle tension, and then we take them through a series of exercises that shows us how their body reacts to stress. Do they react with altered breathing or heart rates? Do they react with muscle tension or cold hands? Do they react through their sweat gland activity? This information helps us understand how they experience stress and what physiological systems in their bodies are more vulnerable. In addition to the psychophysiological stress test, we also use a word-association test to help us understand the psychological vulnerabilities. The unconscious mind often speaks through the body's physiology. We develop a list of twenty words, based on important concepts in the person's life, and see how his or her physiology reacts to those words or concepts. In the list there will be several innocuous words, such as "telephone book" and "paper clip," and other words that are more emotionally loaded, such as "mother," "father," "siblings," "job," "children," and "spouse." Often a person's body is nonresponsive to the innocuous words but very responsive to the emotionally loaded words. For example, when we say "baseball" or "train," there may be no movement in the physiological measurements; but when we say "mother," we often get significant change. If "mother" is a positive emotional construct, then we see the physiology change in a positive way—heart and breathing rates slow, muscles become more relaxed, and hands become warmer and drier. If "mother" is associated with painful or stressful memories, we see the physiology change in a negative way—heart and breathing rates escalate, muscles become more tense, hands become colder, and sweat activity increases.

Angus came to see us for insomnia and headaches. It was clear he was filled with anxiety, which seemed to begin after he was assigned to a new supervisor at work in a local mortgage loan office. He said his boss was controlling, negative, and erratic. His response to the word-association test was dramatic. To all of the words but one he responded in a typical way. Yet the word "supervisor" caused such a negative physiological reaction we were afraid for Angus's health. His heart rate raced, his breathing stopped, his hands became ice cold and very wet, and his muscle tension skyrocketed. If Angus didn't absolutely need his job, we would have encouraged him to quit. Quitting, however, was not an option for Angus. When we showed him how his body reacted to the word "supervisor," he was determined to work through his "boss" issue so that his boss would not affect his physical and emotional health. Using biofeedback, we taught him to become very relaxed and gain tremendous self-control over how his body reacted to stress. We taught him diaphragmatic breathing techniques, as well as hand warming and deep muscle relaxation. In addition, after he learned these self-calming techniques we would stress him with thoughts of his boss and have him imagine negative work interactions while remaining calm. We taught him how to be more effective in dealing with difficult people (his boss). Over time, Angus felt more relaxed at work and started to enjoy the fact that he could have self-control over his physiology no matter what kind of day his boss was having. His moods, muscle tension, and overall well-being were no longer tied to his boss's mood or behavior.

Diaphragmatic Breathing

In our experience, diaphragmatic breathing is the core biofeedback technique. It is simple to teach and, once practiced, simple to implement. Like brain activity, breathing is essential to life and is involved in everything you do. Breathing delivers oxygen from the atmosphere into your lungs, where your blood supply picks it up and takes it to every cell in your body because the cells need it in order to function properly. Breathing also allows you to eliminate waste products, such as carbon dioxide, to keep your internal environment healthy. Too much carbon dioxide causes feelings of disorientation and panic. Brain cells are particularly sensitive to oxygen; they start to die within four minutes when deprived of oxygen. Slight changes in oxygen content in the brain can alter the way a person feels and behaves. When a person gets angry, breathing becomes more shallow and its rate increases significantly (see the illustrations on the next page). This inefficient breathing pattern causes the oxygen content in the angry person's blood to decrease while toxic carbon dioxide waste products increase. Subsequently, the oxygen/carbon dioxide balance is upset, causing irritability, impulsiveness, confusion, and poor decision making.

Learning how to direct and control your breathing has several immediate benefits. It calms the basal ganglia, which controls anxiety; helps the brain run more efficiently; relaxes muscles; warms hands; and regulates the heart's rhythms. We often teach our patients to become experts at breathing slowly, deeply, and from their bellies. Our offices have some very sophisticated biofeedback equipment that uses strain gauges to measure breathing activity. One gauge is placed around a person's chest and a second one around his belly. The equipment measures the movement of the chest and belly as the person breathes in and out. Men especially breathe exclusively with their chests, which is inefficient. If you watch babies or puppies breathe, you will notice that they breathe almost solely with their bellies. That is the most efficient way to breathe.

Expanding your belly when you inhale flattens the diaphragm, pulling the lungs downward and increasing the amount of air available to your lungs and body. Pulling your belly in when you exhale causes the diaphragm to push the air out of your lungs, allowing a more fully exhaled breath, which once again encourages deep breathing. In biofeedback, patients are taught to breathe with their bellies by watching their breathing patterns on a computer screen. In twenty to thirty minutes, most people can learn how to change their breathing patterns, which relaxes them and gives them better control over how they feel and behave.

Here are several simple illustrations to help you understand the anatomy of healthy and unhealthy breathing.

Breathing anatomy

Healthy breathing anatomy during inhalation (flattening the diaphragm and expanding lung capacity)

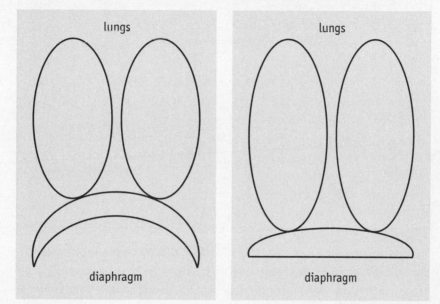

The diaphragm is a bell-shaped muscle that separates the chest cavity and abdomen. When most people breathe in, they don't flatten their diaphragm, which means they aren't using their lungs to full capacity and they have to work harder. By moving your belly out when you inhale, you flatten your diaphragm and significantly increase lung capacity, which calms all body systems.

Few people have access to sophisticated biofeedback equipment, so try the following exercise on your own: Lie on your back and place a small book on your belly. When you inhale, make the book go up; when you exhale, make the book go down. Shifting the energy of breathing lower in your body helps you feel more relaxed and in better control of yourself. You can use this breathing technique to gain greater focus and control over your temper. It is easy to learn and can also be applied to help with sleep and anxiety issues. Another breathing tip: Whenever you feel anxious, mad, or tense, take a deep breath, hold it for four to five seconds, then slowly blow it out (take about six to eight seconds to blow it out). Then take another deep breath, as deep as you can, hold it for four to five seconds, and again

Breathing while angry

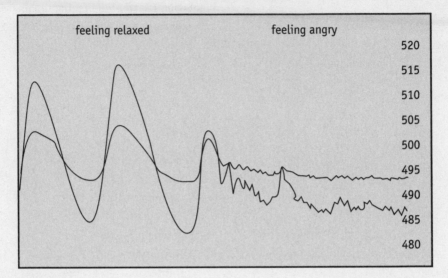

The large waveform is a measurement of abdominal, or belly, breathing by a gauge attached around the belly; the smaller waveform is a measurement of chest breathing by a gauge attached around the upper chest. At rest, this person breathes mostly with his belly (a good pattern), but when he becomes angry his breathing pattern deteriorates, markedly decreasing the oxygen to his brain (common to anger outbursts). No wonder people who have anger outbursts often seem irrational!

slowly blow it out. Do this about ten times and the odds are that you will start to feel very relaxed, if not a little sleepy.

Forty-five-year-old Marie came for evaluation for problems with anxiety and muscle tension. During her first session we noticed that she talked very rapidly and breathed in shallow, quick breaths. We recommended four sessions of breathing biofeedback. She was astonished at how easy diaphragmatic breathing is to learn and how relaxed she could make herself in a short period of time. She quickly noticed that her anxiety improved and she was less tense.

> *Dr. Amen: I have used this technique myself for fifteen years, whenever I feel anxious, angry, stressed, or when I have trouble falling asleep. It sounds so simple, but breathing is essential to life and when we slow down and become more efficient at it, most things seem better. I have scanned myself on a number of occasions. My*

own SPECT scans reveal that my basal ganglia work overtime, indeed, my "hot" basal ganglia fit with my life. As I have said, I tend to be anxious, I want to please others, I bite my fingernails when I'm tense or watching a close ball game, and I have to fight off the fortune-telling ANTs. When I breathe diaphragmatically, my basal ganglia calm down, helping me feel less stress and greater peace within.

Find a Practitioner

In order to use biofeedback effectively, you need to consult with a biofeedback practitioner who understands your particular problem and can train you to get control of it. We recommend practitioners who are certified by the Biofeedback Certification Institute of America. Others may have some knowledge or expertise, but there is no way of telling how much. You are assured that a certified practitioner has at least a minimum level of education and demonstrated ability to help people using biofeedback. You can search for a certified biofeedback practitioner in your area on the Biofeedback Certification Institute of America website at *www.bcia.org*. You can get more information on biofeedback by going to the website for the Association for Applied Psychophysiology and Biofeedback (*www.aapb.org*).

CHAPTER 13

Gender Differences in Anxiety and Depression

The experience of anxiety and depression is the same for men and women in many ways. Fifty percent of those who experience an episode of anxiety and/or depression will have another episode within five years, and many will develop chronic relapsing forms of the disorder. In that case, being male or female doesn't change the risk. Men and women with anxiety disorders or depression also share the tendency to have complicating, or comorbid, conditions. The risk of suicide and suicide attempts is higher for both depressed men and women.

There are a few differences in the course and experience of depression and anxiety that may be gender-related. Women are more likely to have more rapid cycling mood disturbances. Men usually have higher rates of substance abuse and alcoholism as comorbid conditions. An interesting exception is that young women with rapid cycling mood conditions also have high rates of alcohol abuse. Women make more suicide attempts but men usually complete suicide more often. There are growing reports, however, that because women are using increasingly violent methods, their suicide rate is increasing. Women may also have a tendency to have more atypical symptoms of depression, such as weight gain, increased appetite, and excessive sleep.

The most impressive difference between men and women becomes apparent at puberty. In childhood, the rates of anxiety and depression are similar for boys and girls. This begins to change as children reach adolescence. The rate of depression and anxiety among girls begins to rise at puberty and accelerates through the teenage years. Women are diagnosed with anxiety and depression far more commonly than men. Some studies indicate that as many as 15 to 20 percent of women may be suffering from depression. To explain this male-female discrepancy, theories abound ranging from socioeconomic issues to biochemical differences between the sexes.

The sociology and psychology literature provides some intriguing information about the impact of marital status on women's mental health. In general, marriage is correlated to unhappiness for women and happiness for men. Married women with children usually report the highest level of physical and emotional stress symptoms. On the other hand, single women and married men enjoy the highest level of life satisfaction. Single men are not quite as unhappy as married women, and their life satisfaction usually improves when they marry. This is true even for the elderly, according to a recent study reported in the geriatric literature.

Several recent studies have addressed the fact that gender research is biased because it does not control for factors such as socioeconomic conditions and social roles. A May 2002 study conducted in Britain compared men and women working similar jobs in three different organizations: a bank, a university, and the civil service. When the researchers involved in this very large study of 9,988 young men and women controlled for domestic and socioeconomic factors, they found that only in the civil service did the rate of minor psychiatric diagnoses in women exceed that for men to a degree that reached statistical significance. They concluded that generalizations about gender differences might not be helpful because they might vary depending on the context of the study.

Based on our own extensive experience, we believe that both positions have merit. It is true that the majority of medical research is biased in that it does not compare men and women who are working in similar positions, living at similar socioeconomic levels, and operating under similar environmental stress loads. Women are often excluded from drug trials because of the possibility of pregnancy and therefore treatment protocols are optimized for men. We also believe that the rate of anxiety and depression is higher for women than men because there are groups of women who are particularly vulnerable to the development of these illnesses. For example, women who have been abused, those with a history of difficulty at times of hormonal transitions (pregnancy, onset of menses, menopause, and so forth), and those who have undiagnosed ADHD are at higher risk.

Women and Anxiety and Depression

Hormonal Factors

The brains of men and women are organized and operate differently. Sex hormones (especially testosterone and estrogen) are responsible for these structural and functional differences. These hormones act on their receptors in the brain of a developing fetus and cause the structural patterns and circuits to form that are uniquely male or female. Most of us involved in brain research believe that the early influence of the sex hormones accounts for many of the early developmental differences we see in children. For instance, girls usually acquire verbal skills sooner than boys, and boys are generally more physically active than girls.

The sex hormones continue to exert their influence on a person's brain and body during the course of growth and development. These later hormonal effects are called "activational" influences. Activational influences trigger the metamorphosis of a child's body into an adult's. This process starts at puberty and continues through middle adolescence. The physical characteristics and body changes that are produced are called "secondary sex characteristics." There are emotional and mental process changes that occur during adolescence as well. Most women think differently than most men. Women are generally relationship-oriented; they look for group consensus when making decisions, and they form attachments easily and support each other effectively. Men, by nature, tend to be more confrontational than women and more direct or forceful in their communication style; they are less likely to seek help for emotional problems, and are more aggressive in most of their pursuits. These differences in thinking and communication styles are shaped to some extent by the activational effects of hormones.

The cyclic nature of hormonal changes becomes an issue for women at the time of puberty. Hormonal changes occur on a monthly, daily, and moment-to-moment basis. Estrogen and progesterone are the hormones most responsible for regulating a woman's ovarian function, and they exert powerful changes in a woman's body. Estrogen and progesterone play primary roles in supporting the development of secondary sex characteristics, initiating and maintaining menstrual cycles, supporting pregnancy and childbirth, and supplying the protective antioxidant effects and longevity factors that account for women's longer lifespan relative to men's.

We think that these and other powerful hormones are at work in the brain producing neurochemical changes, and some women are more sensitive to these changes than others.

Premenstrual Syndrome

Premenstrual syndrome, while very real, is a much-maligned diagnosis. Unfortunately, it has become a joke and a pejorative term. Bumper stickers proclaiming "I may have cramps, but I can still kill you" attest to this, and most women have had a man in her life comment, "Are you sure you're not just hormonal?" when things aren't going well in the relationship. This prejudice hurts women who truly have a disorder that cycles monthly in relation to their menstrual periods because it implies that the problem is "all in their heads" or is purely emotional.

The psychiatric community has added to the confusion about PMS by repeatedly changing its name. PMS had its name changed to Late Luteal Phase Dysphoric Disorder (LLPDD) and subsequently to Premenstrual Dysphoric Disorder (PMDD). We don't really like LLPDD or PMDD because each implies that dysphoria (profound sadness) is a necessary symptom of the disorder and not everyone has it. Some women have anxiety or are burdened more by physical symptoms than by sadness and depression. We don't necessarily like PMS any better because of the negative press the term gets, but since it is the name by which most women and general practitioners call the disorder, it is the one we use by default.

Statistically, PMS affects 2.5 to 8 percent of women. To meet the diagnostic criteria, the symptoms must begin during the luteal phase of a woman's cycle (day twelve to twenty-eight), and intensify or worsen by at least 30 percent during this phase and resolve with menses. PMS symptoms include mood, behavioral, and physical complaints. The symptoms must also be severe enough to impair the woman's ability to function socially or occupationally. Having a woman chart the nature and severity of her symptoms in relation to her menstrual cycle for three months helps to diagnose PMS.

If a woman's mother or sister has PMS, she is at increased risk of having the disorder. Another significant risk factor is emotional instability or sensitivity at hormonal transition times. If a woman tried to take birth control pills or hormone replacement and didn't tolerate them because they made her sad or irritable, or they gave her a lot of physical side effects, she may be at risk at other hormonal transition times. Women who have a personal or family history of postpartum depression and those who have poor nutrition and exercise patterns are also at higher risk for PMS.

What causes PMS? During the luteal phase of the menstrual cycle, estrogen levels decline and progesterone levels rise dramatically. For women who are hormonally sensitive, this change in hormone levels may be the catalyst for the neuropsychiatric chain of reactions that occurs in their brains.

Many women have heard Dr. Routh lecture on women's issues and have learned about the hormonally driven, brain-based reasons for their emotional fluctuations. Others have come to our clinics and presented us with carefully documented charts of behavioral, emotional, and physical symptoms correlating to their menstrual cycles. Still others come to us with symptoms and are dismayed when their partner voices the belief that the symptoms are directly related to their menstrual cycles. We have a series of brain SPECT images of patients with PMS that were performed during both symptomatic and non-symptomatic times in their cycles. It is the basis for our knowing that PMS is definitely brain-based and biological in nature.

The treatment of PMS involves first making sure that thyroid function is normal. Then the PMS prescription for health requires most women to make a lifestyle change. Most women eat very poorly and women with PMS are no different from other women in this regard. Women with PMS should eat five small meals a day, and each meal should be made up of quality protein and a small amount of complex carbohydrates. This means every meal should include some lean meat, fish, poultry, small amounts of unsalted nuts, eggs, nonfat yogurt, or cottage cheese. A complex carbohydrate should be added, which means half a cup of green beans, one slice of whole wheat bread (not white bread or any other kind), half a cup of broccoli, or one-quarter cup of whole wheat pasta or brown rice. Salads made with leafy vegetables should also be added, but avoid creamy dressings; use balsamic vinegars and vinaigrettes instead. Stay away from potatoes, white bread, pastas, corn, starchy vegetables, beans, most cheeses, cereals, and sweets. These foods turn to sugar as soon as you eat them and make you feel lousy as your blood sugar bounces around. Women with PMS should decrease their consumption of alcohol, caffeine, and carbonated beverages as well.

It helps to know yourself and your particular cycle so that you can manage it most effectively. Knowing that particular times are likely to be more difficult than others allows you to plan for them. Schedule your most important activities at better times in your cycle, plan self-care activities for the more stressful times, and communicate effectively with your support group when you don't feel well. Self-care during the more stressful times in your cycle can mean devoting additional time to simple relaxation, meditation, aromatherapy, getting a massage, or spending additional time with friends. Think about making fitness a part of your life. Even mild to moderate exercise such as walking is beneficial for bloating and fatigue.

When the symptoms of PMS are significant enough that a woman goes to a doctor for help, she usually needs a combination of lifestyle management and medication. Medication is another part of the prescription for health. The most effective treatment available for PMS remains the SSRI medication fluoxetine (Sarafem, Prozac). Some doctors like to give Sarafem or Prozac only during the luteal phase or the days that a woman has symptoms, and other doctors like to give the medication everyday. For women with straightforward PMS, uncomplicated by depression or anxiety disorders, we believe as-needed dosing of Sarafem or Prozac works well. Women who have anxiety or depression complicating their PMS need daily dosing, and, depending on the type of anxiety or depression, they may need other medications as well.

The benzodiazepine Xanax has been used in low doses and on an as-needed dosing schedule during the luteal phase for women who have milder cases of PMS. This seems to work best for women who have complaints of excessive tension and irritability or of high levels of anxiety associated with their PMS. Xanax can be used alone or in combination with Sarafem. The most important management considerations regarding Xanax are that it is potentially addictive, it interacts with alcohol, and it causes drowsiness.

Another part of the prescription for health is the addition of vitamin B-6 50mg twice daily, vitamin C 500 to 1,000mg three times daily, and vitamin E 400 IU twice daily. Oil of Evening Primrose is a naturopathic intervention that has beneficial effects for many women.

Pregnancy and the Postpartum State

Birth, the first and direst of all disasters.
AMBROSE BIERCE (1842–1914)

Pregnancy does not protect women from depression. In fact, at no other time is a woman at greater risk for the onset or relapse of a psychiatric disorder than during pregnancy and the postpartum period. More than one in ten new mothers experience depression after the birth of their baby. Women who have a prior history of depression have an 80 percent chance of experiencing postpartum depression.

The roots of some postpartum issues may be in the myth of the ideal pregnancy, which goes something like this: A woman at her ideal body weight and her partner plan for pregnancy, so she begins taking prenatal vitamins and folic acid at least eight weeks prior to conception. She also stops drinking caffeine and alcohol. Of course, she does not smoke. They conceive their child and she takes absolutely no medications during the course of her pregnancy. Further, she remains perfectly healthy at all times to guard her baby against exposure to viruses, and she gets adequate rest, maintains excellent nutritional status, and continues her fitness program. She happily expects her baby in a stress-free supportive environment, and, after delivering her infant by natural childbirth with no complications, she returns to a caring, loving, and completely supportive environment.

The myth of the ideal pregnancy haunts a lot of women. The reality is that at least 50 percent of all pregnancies are unplanned, 14 percent of deliveries are premature, and 2 to 4 percent of babies are born with severe malformations. Most women are not at their ideal body weight at the time of conception, 80 percent take at least one medication during the course of their pregnancy for some sort of acute or chronic illness, and 33 percent take psychoactive medications. The rate of fetal exposure to alcohol, tobacco, and drugs is increasing, and most women are pregnant before they realize they have exposed their baby. Many women—in fact, most women—do not get through pregnancy without at least a minor complication or scare, and after the first few days following delivery, these new mothers usually find themselves trying to heal and cope with a baby on their own without much help and support. Then the Baby Blues set in.

The Baby Blues affect 85 percent of women. Symptoms begin within the first two weeks after delivery, peak within five days, and usually resolve within ten days. Women with the Baby Blues are tearful and experience anxiety, irritability, and sadness, or sometimes they just feel moody. Baby Blues follow a time-limited, benign course. They respond to support and reassurance from loved ones.

In contrast to the Baby Blues, postpartum depression is a devastating illness that cripples a mother's ability to care for herself and her infant. Postpartum depression strikes at the core of the mother-child relationship by interfering with bonding and attachment, damaging both individuals emotionally. In its most aggressive forms, Bipolar Disorder and depression with psychotic features, postpartum depression has potentially lethal consequences.

Postpartum Depression

Anna, a thirty-one-year-old Hispanic woman, looked exhausted and sat silently in our office. Her husband and mother-in-law explained that Anna had given birth to a healthy baby girl nine months earlier, and, like almost all new mothers, Anna had developed a case of the Baby Blues. She had felt emotionally down and was tearful, and her self-confidence seemed shaken. Anna's mother-in-law had seen this happen to many new mothers and knew it would pass with reassurance and family support. As time went on, Anna grew sadder and lost weight and seemed unable to care for the baby. Anna's obstetrician had urged her to take an antidepressant, but she was breast-feeding and was afraid to take medication. Anna stopped wanting to see any of her friends and could not be talked into going out of the house for any activity because getting dressed was overwhelming for her. Anna began to wonder if her husband still loved her. When the baby cried, Anna was sure that her baby was "better off with its grandmother anyway." When Anna started having suicidal thoughts, her family brought her in for evaluation in spite of her reluctance and hopelessness.

During the resting state, Anna's brain showed deactivation in the prefrontal cortex and markedly increased activity in her limbic system. This explained the low motivation, difficulty planning for activities, inability to concentrate, and profound depression that Anna was feeling. When she concentrated, her SPECT scan showed some improvement in the activity level of the prefrontal cortex but Anna's limbic system remained very active. This pattern showed that Anna's prefrontal cortex was trying to respond to the concentration task but that her limbic system was still limiting her.

Being able to see "proof" of a brain-based reason for her thoughts and feelings allowed Anna to accept treatment for her postpartum depression.

New mothers like Anna remain at increased risk for depression for up to two years after the birth of their baby. Less than one-third of women with postpartum mood disorders seek treatment even when they feel their lives ebbing away and are unable to enjoy the experience of mothering their new baby. Oftentimes family members, friends, and doctors participate in the process of denial and avoidance. They ignore symptoms initially because the symptoms mimic normal pregnancy and postpartum states—decreased self-esteem; fatigue; decreased libido; and changes in appetite, sleep, and energy levels—and later because they mistakenly attribute them to Baby Blues, an adjustment phase, or some other benign condition with equally disastrous potential outcomes.

Untreated anxiety and depression can adversely affect fetal birth weight and gestational age at delivery. Depression, anxiety, and high levels of stress cause increased levels of circulating stress hormones in the mother, and excessive levels of maternal stress hormones affect fetal brain development. When depression or anxiety strikes a female patient, it must be treated aggressively.

Obsessive-Compulsive Disorder

Pregnancy is a very common time for Obsessive-Compulsive Disorder (OCD) to appear. Reportedly, 52 percent of women with OCD experienced the onset during their first pregnancy. This is likely a hormonally mediated effect. Women are extremely disturbed by the symptoms of OCD, which can include thoughts of harming their child, extreme fears of germs contaminating baby food, or unrealistic preoccupations with the health of the child. They may develop elaborate rituals and find themselves excessively washing their baby to remove toxins from its body, or they may feel compelled to spend many hours sterilizing the baby's clothing, toys, and eating utensils to remove germs. The level of anxiety and panic becomes intolerable for many of these women and they may even begin to avoid caring for their children for fear of harming them.

Margo was a thirty-six-year-old elementary schoolteacher who was five months pregnant with her first child when her family doctor referred her for evaluation and treatment. Margo had no prior history of psychiatric treatment. She and her husband were happily expecting their baby and she had been healthy during the pregnancy. During the month prior to her appointment at our clinic, Margo had developed unwanted thoughts and mental images about knives. She described these thoughts and images as "crazy and coming from nowhere." The thoughts and images centered on fears that she would stab her child. As the frequency of the thoughts and disturbing images increased, Margo began to develop rituals to make the thoughts go away. She found a special drawer in her home for all the sharp knives and kept them locked up. Margo needed to count the knives many times during the day, after they were used, and before she went to bed at night to ensure that none was missing. She then became concerned that she would "accidentally" pick up a knife at the school cafeteria or at a restaurant and thereby endanger her future child. As her anxiety level rose, she began to avoid places where she might come in contact with a knife. Margo could not concentrate at work and found herself constantly checking on the knives at home. She was anxious and unable to cope with what she knew were unrealistic fears. When she read a newspaper article about OCD, she recognized the symptoms and called her family doctor, who referred her to us for evaluation.

We weren't able to scan Margo because she was pregnant; instead, we went to our teaching files to show her images of the anterior cingulate gyrus and to explain its role in the genesis of OCD. Margo, like most of our patients, was amazed to see the before-and-after images of OCD sufferers who had been treated with medication. In these cases, symptom reduction was correlated to normalization of activity levels in the anterior cingulate gyrus. She already knew that her thoughts and the disturbing intrusive images were "not real." She didn't think she was crazy and yet the thoughts and behaviors were so unlike her that she sometimes wondered if she was losing her mind. She had never been aggressive or violent but was becoming increasingly worried that she would somehow "lose control and act on the images." Margo had hoped the problem was biological. Now she had evidence that this was the case, and she wanted treatment.

The management of neuropsychiatric disorders during pregnancy and lactation is constantly evolving and there is much that we do not yet know. However, we do know that exposure to untreated maternal illness is more dangerous for a fetus or child than many of our modern medications. We've already noted that increased levels of maternal stress hormones adversely affect fetal brain development and that untreated psychiatric illness in a mother affects fetal birth weight and gestational age at delivery. These are very important concerns. Attachment disorders and disruption of the mother–child bond, behavioral difficulties in the child, and an increased incidence of learning problems are additional consequences of an untreated psychiatric illness in a mother.

We are strong advocates for women's mental health and consequently find ourselves opposing the prevailing opinions of many primary care doctors and psychiatrists who withhold treatment of pregnant and breast-feeding women. We believe these well-meaning physicians are misguided and that in fact women have been misled to believe that treatment of neuropsychiatric disorders is harmful to infants and developing fetuses when in fact exposure to the disorder itself often poses much more risk. As far as we know, most antidepressants pose little risk to a woman or her developing baby during pregnancy and are most likely safe for use during breast-feeding. However, the safest medications are the SSRIs, and of these the most studied drug for use in pregnancy and breast-feeding is Prozac, the original SSRI. Prozac is a very safe medication that has not been associated with any increased risk of pregnancy complications and is safe for breast-feeding babies. There is also a growing body of literature supporting the safety of Wellbutrin for use in pregnancy and breast-feeding, including case reports indicating Wellbutrin could not be detected in the blood of breast-fed babies whose mothers were taking the compound. The other SSRI medications and Effexor have not been associated with any increased problems in babies or mothers but do not yet have as much data supporting their use.

Lithium remains the gold standard for treatment of acute mania, and many women with Bipolar Disorder take lithium for maintenance therapy. Others take it for a variety of other reasons including the treatment of migraine headaches and thyroid conditions and to boost antidepressant response. Pregnant women with a history of mania are frequently started on lithium one to two weeks prior to delivery because of the 80 percent chance that they will relapse in the first two weeks after delivery without treatment. Women already taking lithium need to be carefully monitored because the levels fluctuate widely based on fluid balance and will rapidly become toxic immediately after delivery. They may require frequent dose adjustments. Lithium is one of the medications that uncommonly may affect a developing baby's thyroid gland, heart, and kidneys. It also is excreted in breast milk and can cause symptoms in a baby such as lethargy, tremors, and irritability. For these reasons, the newest recommendations are to switch bipolar women to anticonvulsants (if possible) and to use those anticonvulsants that appear to be the safest or that cross into breast milk the least. The two best anticonvulsant choices meeting these criteria are Lamictal and Depakote. If a pregnant woman or new mother needs an antipsychotic, Clozaril should be avoided because it has caused "floppy infant syndrome." The conventional antipsychotics such as Haldol cause some babies to look sedated or sleepy, and therefore the newer antipsychotics such as Zyprexa may be preferable because of their overall improved safety profile and decreased number of side effects. However, the latter are too new to have been studied extensively in pregnant and breast-feeding women.

The benzodiazepines are often prescribed in combination with antidepressants to treat anxious depressions, OCD, Panic Disorder, and a variety of other complicated psychiatric disorders. They are also prescribed as single agents to treat Restless Legs Syndrome, acute insomnia, and some medical disorders. There are many benzodiazepines available and, of them, Klonopin appears to be a good choice for use in pregnancy. Valium tends to accumulate in babies who are breast-fed and makes them drowsy and lose weight. The short-acting benzodiazepine Restoril, commonly prescribed for insomnia, is another good choice because it is eliminated from the mother's system rapidly and therefore not much is passed on to the baby through breast milk. The American Academy of Pediatrics recommends Ambien, which is a non-benzodiazepine medication for insomnia, because it is rapidly cleared from the mother's system and does not affect the baby.

Finally, full-spectrum light therapy is of benefit to some pregnant women with depression. Just like patients with Seasonal Affective Disorder, pregnant women who are exposed to morning bright-light therapy have symptom reduction, according to a recent study at Yale University. Researchers there found that after three weeks of exposure to bright morning light, sixteen depressed pregnant patients improved by 49 percent with no evidence of side effects. The study was limited by its small size and by the fact that it lasted for a total of only five weeks, but the results are still promising.

Other Anxiety Disorders

Women may be three times more likely than men to have anxiety disorders. Researchers at Henry Ford Hospital in Detroit studied the correlation between women's increased risk of anxiety and their increased risk of depression. More than 1,000 young adults were randomly recruited from a health maintenance organization in southeastern Michigan for the study. The researchers learned that a previous anxiety disorder increases the risk of depression in both sexes, and, interestingly, they learned that women are not more vulnerable than men to depression after a previous anxiety disorder. The importance of this study is that it confirms the link between anxiety and depression (an observation we have independently confirmed through our imaging work). One of the researchers' conclusions was that, since women have a much greater incidence of anxiety disorders, they will logically have a much greater risk of depression.

Posttraumatic Stress Disorder (PTSD) is often conceptualized as an illness that is most likely to affect soldiers who have been involved in combat actions. However, PTSD affects many more women than men. It is under-diagnosed even in female veterans who, when exposed to the same type of stress as their male counterparts, develop the same type of symptoms but are less likely to be correctly diagnosed and treated. Rape trauma, childhood sexual abuse, abusive relationships, breast cancer, pregnancy loss, abortion, and complications during pregnancy and delivery are some of the events that lead to the very high incidence of PTSD in women. For women who have PTSD, pregnancy and labor and delivery can also trigger flashbacks, nightmares, and intrusive thoughts about prior traumatic events.

The treatment protocols for anxiety are the same for pregnant and breast-feeding women as for women who are not pregnant or breast-feeding. We use the SSRI medications like Prozac because of the large body of literature supporting its safety for women and babies, and we also use benzo-diazepines and many of the anticonvulsants we have discussed. Anxiety disorders are also very responsive to biofeedback, EMDR (eye movement desensitization and reprocessing), self-relaxation, and cognitive behavioral interventions.

Perimenopause

I can't remember anything anymore.   CHARLIE BROWN
I can't even remember what I had for lunch.   LINUS
I can't remember what I had for supper.   LUCY
I had dog food.   SNOOPY

Women between the ages of thirty-five and forty-five should think about the conversation above between the Charlie Brown characters. Anyone who can identify with Charlie, Linus, or Lucy may be experiencing one of the most common symptoms of perimenopause—memory dysfunction. Memory trouble, the inability to think clearly, irritability, fatigue, and insomnia are the most common complaints of women in perimenopause.

Perimenopause is a transitional phase leading to menopause during which ovarian function becomes variable and hormone levels begin to fluctuate unpredictably, leading to symptoms that correlate to the rising and falling hormone levels. This transition to menopause usually lasts three to five years but may last as long as ten years. Estrogen levels may rise to very high levels and then fall to extremely low levels, causing the first hot flashes, flushing, and occasional flares of migraine headaches. Progesterone levels also begin to fluctuate and follicle-stimulating hormone levels rise as cycles become unresponsive to this hormone and no eggs are released. Menstrual cycles gradually become more irregular and women who have had PMS problems may have an increase in symptoms at this time.

As perimenopause continues, the symptoms of estrogen withdrawal become more troublesome and women experience a worsening of hot flashes, sweating, and flushing. Fatigue and daytime drowsiness are frequent complaints of women in perimenopause. Insomnia and frequent awakenings throughout the night compound the problem of daytime fatigue.

Women begin to notice the cosmetic effects of lack of estrogen during perimenopause. The skin rapidly loses subcutaneous (below the surface) fat, collagen, and support proteins in the absence of estrogen. Estrogen also helps the skin maintain its water content and elasticity. Estrogen acts on breast tissue to maintain its structure, firmness, and fullness. When estrogen levels decline, women notice an increase in wrinkles and other skin changes such as a coarser appearance, more facial hair, or thinning of their skin. Women also notice that their breasts seem less full or that "gravity has taken over" and they complain of sagging.

Libido and sexual response may also become issues at this time in a woman's life as estrogen withdrawal wreaks havoc in this area as well. Estrogen is vitally necessary for normal sexual response in women, and, as levels decline, women suffer vaginal atrophy and dryness and psychological complications such as decreased sexual desire, lack of arousal, and difficulty achieving orgasm.

Women with a history of anxiety or depression at other hormonally sensitive times, such as during treatment with oral contraceptive pills, treatment for infertility, hormone replacement, pregnancy, the postpartum period, or after pregnancy loss, are at increased risk for recurrence during perimenopause. Women with Attention Deficit Disorder may experience a worsening of their symptoms at this time and may need their medication adjusted.

As always, the evaluation process begins with making sure that a woman does not have a medical condition that could be causing her symptoms, especially a thyroid condition. A woman with depression and anxiety who is also in perimenopause needs both of her conditions treated in order to have a full response. This means we develop a treatment plan that is specific for her type of anxiety and/or depression and refer her to one of our colleagues who specializes in gynecology to coordinate the treatment of her hormonal imbalance. Perimenopausal women need hormone replacement in the form of birth control pills, estrogen replacement, or phytoestrogens (soy protein, flaxseed oil) if the condition is mild.

Perimenopause is a wake-up call for a woman to begin to take care of herself and to advocate for her health—mental, physical, and spiritual. This is not only a hormonal transition time, it is a social and psychological transition time for many women as well. Just as their first wrinkles appear and hot flashes start, many women find themselves facing mounting economic and emotional demands to cope with changes in their family structure. Their children are starting to leave home and their own aging parents need help. Some of these women also face abandonment by their spouses. Most women are shocked to learn that the same insurance companies that pay for Viagra for male sexual dysfunction often won't pay for their birth control pills prescribed for perimenopause or for contraception. To successfully manage these emotional and physical demands, perimenopausal women need to attend to their mental health by having their hormonal and neuropsychiatric conditions, if present, identified and treated. They also need to make a lifelong commitment to their physical health at this time by developing a nutrition and fitness program. As we have said many times, women do not eat well and this is particularly true of women who are facing perimenopause and menopause, when nutritional demands for essential vitamins, minerals, protein, and fatty acids are high. This is the time for women to adopt a quality high-protein, low-carbohydrate diet (see also the PMS section on page 219). A fitness program that incorporates weight lifting and mild to moderate aerobic exercise to increase bone and muscle density is extremely important.

Every woman should take a multivitamin daily. The antioxidants vitamin C 500 to 1,000mg two to three times daily and vitamin E 400 IU twice daily should also be taken. Because hardly anyone gets enough calcium, women should be taking this as well and the one to look for is USP elemental or precipitated calcium. Perimenopausal women should take 1,000 to 1,500mg daily.

Don't neglect spirituality, either. Make room in your life for the things that renew your soul and restore your spirit. Make time for the activities and people that balance you, bring you comfort, and nurture you. Practice and explore the arts, sciences, religions, and languages that expand your mind.

Menopause

Menopause is defined as the absence of menses for one year and most American women enter menopause at 51.4 years of age. Menopause is caused by the rather abrupt withdrawal from a woman's system of the very potent estrogen estradiol, as ovarian function ceases. There are many bothersome symptoms that herald the withdrawal of estrogen, including hot flashes, mood disturbance, weight gain, night sweats, fatigue, and sleep disturbance. These are not simply annoying symptoms, nor are they peripheral effects of hormone loss; they are warning signals that brain function is disturbed by the absence of estrogen. Sleep is regulated by the brain, and in the absence of estrogen a woman in menopause may have her sleep disturbed every fifteen seconds to eighteen minutes. The hypothalamus reacts to a lack of estrogen by causing engorgement or dilation of blood vessels, which results in hot flashes.

Evidence is mounting that lack of estrogen is bad for the brain. This discovery began with rat studies. Rats that have their ovaries removed have a huge estrogen deficit just like menopausal women. Estrogen-deficit rats have trouble learning, and they have deterioration of their temporal lobes, the area of the brain that is responsible for learning and memory. When rats were given estrogen replacement, the number of connections between cells in their temporal lobes improved, and so did their ability to learn new tasks. There have since been many studies showing the same pattern in human females. Women who have undergone surgical removal of their ovaries or who have gone through natural menopause often have difficulty with memory, concentration, and attention span. They have more trouble learning skills, they have more word-finding difficulty, and they feel overwhelmed by complex tasks that were previously easily mastered. These same women have marked and rapid reversal of these symptoms with estrogen replacement.

SPECT and PET scans of postmenopausal women who have not taken estrogen replacement show deactivation of the prefrontal cortex and temporal lobes. Neuropsychological testing of these women indicates impaired cognitive functioning in the areas of attention span, concentration, and learning. When these women are treated with estrogen replacement therapy or Evista, a selective estrogen receptor modulator, their performance on testing markedly improved. Of great interest, the SPECT and PET scans of the treated women also showed greatly improved brain function.

Researchers followed a group of 2,000 women over age sixty-five for three years to examine the relationship between cognitive function and hormone replacement. Their results were published in the medical journal *Neurology* and showed that hormone replacement had positive mental performance benefits for women and that the oldest women benefited most of all.

The evidence is mounting that women who take hormone replacement have a significantly reduced risk of Alzheimer's disease, perhaps as great as 60 percent. While there is no evidence that estrogen will stop the progression of Alzheimer's once it has started, many researchers believe that estrogen is protective against the onset of the illness. Estrogen is a powerful antioxidant and neutralizes free radicals that damage brain cells during the aging process. It also helps prevent the formation of plaques that characterize Alzheimer's disease.

Lack of estrogen over time causes osteoporosis. Without estrogen your bones become progressively thinner or more porous, placing you at increasingly greater risk of fractures. By the age of eighty, an average woman who has not taken hormone replacement will lose four inches in height because of vertebral compression fractures. Her spine literally crumbles over time and may cause chronic pain. Twenty-five to 50 percent of women like her, who have been in untreated menopause for more than twenty-five years, will suffer a debilitating hip fracture, and only one in three of those who do will make a full recovery. Estrogen deficiency increases the risk of bladder problems, colon cancer, and the biggest killer of women—cardiovascular disease.

As if all that weren't enough, lack of estrogen makes your skin wrinkle and the connective tissue layers beneath your skin break down, so it sags. Meanwhile your metabolism changes, and your bones and muscles atrophy or shrink from lack of estrogen so you lose muscle mass and pack on more fat. Libido frequently diminishes and so does sexual response because estrogen is necessary for normal sexual functioning. Testosterone is important for women just as it is for men, and as ovarian function continues to deteriorate, less testosterone is available. Lack of testosterone further decreases sexual responsiveness and interest.

Menopause represents a time of increased risk for women who have previously experienced the onset of anxiety or depression during other hormonal transition periods. Women who became emotionally sensitive while taking birth control pills, or who had a postpartum depression, or who suffered from PMS are among those at increased risk of another episode during menopause. Anxiety and depression may be inadequately treated and are not always recognized in menopausal women because the symptoms are mistaken for those of menopause itself or because they are falsely thought to be an adjustment phase to menopause. Sudden flashes of body heat, sweating, and shakiness could be erroneously thought to be panic attacks. When complaints of trouble with memory, concentration, sleep patterns, fatigue, weight gain, and moodiness are voiced, they sound very much like depression.

How do we know our patient has symptoms of menopause, anxiety, depression, or all of these? We start with a very careful interview of the patient. Laboratory tests help if we still have questions, and so does a referral to one of our colleagues in gynecology. And one of our most powerful tools is our ability to image the brain. A brain deprived of one of the basic substances it needs for optimal functioning has a characteristic pattern, and if depression and/or anxiety is complicating matters, we will see evidence of that as well.

Our approach to menopause is straightforward. We are strong advocates for women and believe that all aspects of women's health must be addressed. This has never been truer than now, as women can expect to live thirty or more years beyond menopause. Treating the whole woman means providing her with all the information available to protect her brain and to optimize her general fitness level. The treatment of anxiety and depression has been extensively covered in this book and in most aspects is the same at menopause as it is at other times in a woman's life. Some medications need to be started at lower doses and increased more slowly for older women. Older people tend to be on more medications than younger people and therefore physicians need to pay attention to potential drug interactions.

Even when appropriate medications and therapy are applied for the treatment of psychiatric conditions, depression and anxiety symptoms may not fully respond without hormone replacement therapy. And we strongly advocate hormone replacement for any healthy menopausal woman to protect her brain and to promote good brain functioning and body health. Many women reading this will be apprehensive because of the confusion caused by the recently released data concerning participants in the Women's Health Initiative (WHI) who were using Prempro, a medication that contains a combination of estrogen and progesterone. The study was stopped after 5.2 years because researchers found that some women in the study had a higher risk of breast cancer, strokes, blood clots, and heart attacks. This announcement caused many women to abruptly stop hormone therapy and raised the anxiety level of those who chose to continue taking estrogen.

We have reservations about the WHI trial. The trial treated all women with the same medication, Prempro, and with the same dose. We believe that hormone therapy must be individualized for each woman, just like any other medication we recommend. Every woman must be carefully evaluated for underlying risk factors for the development of cancers, heart disease, and blood clots. It is not clear that this was adequately done in the WHI study. The WHI reported only relative rather than absolute risks during hormone therapy. In other words, the risk for any given woman is very, very small. The results of this trial can be applied only to Prempro users and not to hormone replacement in general. Groups of researchers who used different forms of estrogen and progestins than Prempro have reported no increase in heart attacks in their trials. Lending more support for the need to individualize treatment is the belief of many practitioners that it is the form of progestin used, and not estrogen, that increases a woman's risk of breast cancer.

The message we want to convey is that hormone therapy is safe when it is individualized and closely supervised. Women derive great benefit in terms of quality of life when they take hormone replacement.

Women who have a history of breast cancer or significant risk factors have the option of taking Evista (raloxifene), a selective estrogen receptor modulator that has reduced the risk of breast cancer by up to 70 percent in some studies. Some women who have been taking standard hormone replacement (estrogens and progestins) for longer than a decade develop a slightly increased risk of breast cancer and they, too, are candidates to switch to Evista.

Women in menopause should pay excellent attention to their diet and fitness level. A high-quality protein diet and a weight-lifting program to preserve muscle mass and bone strength are more important at this time of life than ever. Antioxidants should be started or continued if you are already taking them. The antioxidants are vitamin C 500 to 1,000mg two to three times daily and vitamin E 400 IU twice daily. Of course, estrogen is the most powerful antioxidant known. A multivitamin should be taken every day and women between the ages of fifty-one and seventy should take vitamin D 400 IU, and after age seventy-one the dose should be increased to 600 IU.

Calcium intake is important and hardly anyone gets enough in their diet. Menopausal women need 1,500 to 2,000mg every day, so consider a supplement for this as well. The type of calcium is important, so check labels. Look for USP formulations of elemental or precipitated calcium. If you have risk factors for osteoporosis (you are a smoker, weigh less than 127 pounds, are Caucasian or Asian, have a family history of osteoporosis, are past menopause or have had a hysterectomy and are not on HRT, do not exercise, have a poor diet, abuse alcohol, use steroids for asthma, or have thyroid disease) or you have any reason to believe you are experiencing bone loss, you should immediately seek the opinion of a specialist for advice. You may benefit from a bone scan and you may need treatment with calcitonin, Fosamax, and other medications to protect your bones. At the time of the writing of this book, Eli Lilly and Company, the manufacturer of Evista, has a parathyroid hormone preparation in clinical trials that looks very promising for the treatment of osteoporosis, especially when used in combination with hormone replacement therapy. Parathyroid hormone helps women rebuild bone density. For more information, go to the company's website, *www.Lilly.com,* and check on hPTH1-34.

If you do not have a substance abuse problem, a glass of red wine every day is beneficial. Taking ibuprofen 200mg daily with food may decrease the risk of Alzheimer's disease. The cyclooxygenase inhibitor Vioxx appears to be even more effective but cost may be a limiting factor for most people. The antioxidants, hormone replacement, and exercise that we have recommended in the preceding paragraphs help boost memory and brain performance by increasing oxygenation and circulation. Phosphatidylserine 100mg three times daily, Siberian ginseng 100 to 200mg daily, and a vitamin B-complex taken daily may also be beneficial for brain health. Ginkgo biloba 80mg three times daily is also helpful but has the unwanted side effect of acting as a blood thinner and should be avoided at least three weeks prior to and after surgery. Dihydroepiandrosterone (DHEA) and testosterone should also be considered for postmenopausal and perimenopausal women who are taking hormone replacement.

Unrecognized/Undertreated ADD

We have devoted years of our lives to the study of ADD. Through our efforts to refine and improve diagnosis and treatment of ADD and to educate others about our work, we have recognized a large population of unrecognized and undertreated cases. We are not alone in this observation. Many other researchers and clinicians have also taken note of this group that is, for the most part, made up of females. The ADD cases that are most easily missed are the inattentive subtypes, the ones that do not have associated hyperactivity, and this is the variant most commonly seen in females.

The inattentive ADD patient tends to look like a daydreamer or a slow learner. She does not disrupt class, but often has poor follow-through and low motivation, and she seems internally preoccupied. She is at risk of getting patted on the head and told that she doesn't need to learn math because girls aren't usually as good at it as boys are anyway. Her parents hope that she'll marry someone capable of providing a good living because she didn't do well enough in school to predict job success for herself. This is very unfortunate because the inattentive form of ADD is very responsive to treatment.

No matter what form of ADD a woman has, and certainly many girls are hyperactive, ADD gets worse at hormonal transition times. This is particularly true of untreated ADD. The worsening symptoms with which ADD women struggle at perimenopause, menopause, during the postpartum period, and when PMS is very bad are most likely due to low estrogen levels. Lack of estrogen causes difficulty with concentration, fatigue, poor energy regulation, and memory dysfunction. These estrogen deficiency–generated cognitive problems compound ADD symptoms. Women who are already being treated for ADD may need to have their medications adjusted. Women not previously diagnosed with ADD may experience worsening of their symptoms at hormonal transition times and may require treatment.

The Sexist Diseases

The sexist illnesses are those that preferentially affect women. Some common examples are fibromyalgia, CFS, migraine headaches, some forms of arthritis, varicose and spider veins, thyroid disorders, and systemic lupus erythematosus. Many women notice that their condition flares at predictable times in their menstrual cycle or at hormonal transition times. This is not surprising since we know that estrogen affects neurotransmitter systems. When estrogen levels are stable, serotonin transmission is enhanced. Conversely, when estrogen levels are low, women with migraine conditions are more prone to headaches. This mechanism may apply to many other illnesses as well.

Women with chronic pain conditions are also prone to depression and anxiety disorders. They may benefit from treatment with a combination of antidepressants (SSRIs or Serzone) and hormone therapy.

Sexual Dysfunction

Women's sexuality is the dark continent of the soul.

SIGMUND FREUD (1856–1939)

At least four in ten American women experience some form of sexual dissatisfaction, according to most surveys and studies that we have read. A quick glance at the feature articles of the top-selling magazines would lead you to believe the numbers are much higher.

There are four distinct types of sexual disorders that affect women: lack of desire or low libido, problems with arousal, inability to achieve orgasm or difficulty achieving orgasm, and pain that is associated with intercourse. The first step in treating sexual disorders that affect women is to identify and treat any medical problems that may be causing the problem. Pelvic surgery or injuries, untreated high blood pressure and heart disease, diabetes, infections, and smoking are all examples of medical conditions that cause pain, decreased sensation, and difficulty with arousal. Hormonal problems such as lack of estrogen and testosterone after menopause, thyroid disorders, postpartum conditions, and other less common endocrine abnormalities such as pituitary tumors impair sexual response and decrease sexual interest. Commonly prescribed medications also create sexual side effects and these include the antidepressants, blood pressure medications, ulcer medications, seizure medications, birth control pills, and many others.

After treating any underlying medical conditions and/or medication side effects, the next step is to look for psychiatric conditions that need attention. Low libido can obviously be a symptom of depression and should improve as depression lifts. However, as we've already discussed, it can also be a side effect of medications that we use to treat depression. PTSD is extremely common in women. The most common cause of head injuries in women is physical abuse by men with whom they live—husbands, fathers, and boyfriends. Women are also victimized by rape and sexual abuse at appallingly high rates. For a woman with a history of abuse of any sort, the stage is set for the development of PTSD, other anxiety disorders, self-esteem problems, and the inability to respond sexually to her partner because of shame and fear. Substance abuse and promiscuity are other ways that women with past histories of rape and sexual abuse sometimes cope with the events.

The overwhelming pressure that women face today is another factor that must not be overlooked. The vast majority of women, including mothers, work. Even though they have a partner, married mothers do essentially the same amount of housework and child care as do single mothers. It is therefore not surprising that on surveys married women with children rate themselves as the least happy and healthy people, and single women rate themselves as the happiest and healthiest. Married men rank themselves just slightly below the single women, and single men are the only ones who think they are as miserable as married women with children. The working mother earns less than her male counterparts although she does the same job and has the same education. She then comes home to housework and child care. At the end of her day she is exhausted and does not experience sexual activity with her partner as something she is doing for herself, but rather as "one more thing she has to do for someone else." This feeling is most often because of lack of passion.

Not to put one more burden on women's shoulders, but women have to take charge of their sexuality. This means taking greater responsibility for knowing what gives them pleasure and communicating it to their partners. Women often assume that men know how to set romantic moods and be wonderful lovers. Unfortunately, men are often clueless about what women want. Think about the setting that works best for you, and if you need candlelight, mirrors, and a massage, tell your partner. If telling your partner how to touch you is too difficult, use body language to communicate with him. Move his hand or reposition him to change the rhythm of your lovemaking. Remember that men did not come into the world with a "how to give sexual pleasure to women" handbook. If you read something you like, hand it to your man; men are usually very interested to know what satisfies a woman sexually.

So, what if you're with the most passionate, sexually fulfilling man in the world and still find yourself having problems? We start with our checklist and rule out medical causes, such as thyroid conditions, diabetes, substance abuse, and several other medical illnesses that we've already discussed in detail. Then we look for depression and anxiety as a cause for the problem and treat those accordingly. We also pay attention to medications that may be causing sexual dysfunction, and of course there are many, including some that we use to treat anxiety and depression. We discuss sexual side effects of psychiatric medications in detail in chapter 7. Many other medications that cause sexual dysfunction need to be evaluated in terms of dosage, elimination, or switching to another compound that doesn't cause the problem.

Finally, sexual dysfunction that doesn't respond to other interventions may respond to treatment with Wellbutrin, an antidepressant that has pro-sexual effects. Wellbutrin is more fully discussed in chapter 7. Viagra is also being prescribed for women with increasing frequency and has been helpful for a number of them, and in many cases testosterone therapy in the form of creams that are applied topically is of benefit to women who are meno-pausal or perimenopausal.

Thoughts for Men

Men may have somewhat lower rates of anxiety and depression than women. We use the word "may" because we believe some traditional male personal-ity traits are shifting the statistics. One of these classic male characteristics is denial. Denial is an adaptive mechanism that is generally more highly devel-oped in men than in women. Like any other personality trait or psycholog-ical mechanism, denial is not a bad thing when used appropriately. For instance, denial allows people to set aside their immediate needs and focus on larger or more urgent issues at hand. It is what allows soldiers to ignore pain and to continue defending themselves and those around them; police officers and firefighters to risk personal injury and loss of life to save the lives of citizens; nurses and doctors to continue working long hours caring for sick and injured people; and mothers and fathers to tirelessly care for babies at night. However, this same altruistic trait can get people into trouble when it is applied to the wrong situations. Men have a much greater level of de-nial of illness than women, and when they are willing to admit to a prob-lem, men often delay seeking help and then are more resistant to treatment than women. Because our society puts such a premium on male strength and virility, men often view any admission of a problem or illness as weakness or, even more significantly, as evidence of loss of manhood. Men are socialized differently, too. Little girls talk openly about emotions; they are allowed to show a full range of emotions and girls and women freely touch each other supportively. By contrast, little boys learn quickly to suppress tears, that laughter and aggression are the only emotions allowed, that touching other males is off-limits unless during sports or aggression, and that talking about emotions will get them labeled a "sissy."

There are also differences in the ways in which anxiety and depression are experienced by men and women, and these differences may influence how and when the symptoms are reported. For instance, men have much higher rates of alcohol and drug dependence associated with depression and this could mask a higher rate of depression in men. Men, more often than women, manage their feelings, especially anxiety and depression, by acting out. Acting-out behaviors are self-destructive and lead men impulsively into high-risk situations and to thoughtlessly consume to excess whatever is immediately available. Acting-out behaviors take the form of sexual addiction and high-risk sexual behavior, aggression against others, and substance abuse and crime to support the habit. It also means drinking to cope with stress, avoiding communication with your partner, breaking things around the house when you are angry, and verbally abusing people. Men who act out are the drivers who impulsively chase people who accidentally cut them off in traffic. They drive at excessive speeds, engage in high-risk sports, and don't take care of injuries. Acting out also means abusing one's self in ways such as overeating, ignoring health care (not taking insulin if you are diabetic), or smoking.

Acting-out behaviors are often forms of denial or attempts to self-medicate underlying psychiatric conditions such as anxiety and depression. They account for the very high rates of head injuries in men. The increased rates of ADD, substance abuse, impulse-control disorders, and Antisocial Personality Disorder also increase the risk of head injuries in men. Head injuries very commonly have depressive symptoms associated with them that are easily missed.

We also know that there are brain-based reasons for male-female differences in the experience and reporting of symptoms of anxiety and depression. Under the influence of the sex hormones (estrogen and testosterone), the developing brain lays down structural patterns and circuits that cause it to be female or male in nature. Male brains are lateralized, or one-sided, for many cognitive functions. Females tend to use both sides of their brain more often and this access to both hemispheres of the brain may be the origin of "women's intuition." Because men tend to have more left-sided dominance, they tend to be more direct and "to the point." They are less likely to recognize emotional issues, less likely to discuss a problem at length, and less likely to recognize a condition early.

Men also commit suicide at much higher rates than women. This is likely a function of their lack of recognition of problems in the early stages combined with denial. It may also be a bonding and attachment issue. Adult men have less activity in their limbic system, and one of the functions of the limbic system is bonding and attachment. Very depressed men may commit suicide at higher rates because they are less relationship-oriented than women. If they do not feel strongly bonded and attached to a peer group, community, or family, they are unlikely to consider the impact of suicide on those left behind.

Fortunately, we are able to treat many men in our clinic because we treat their children. Some men who bring their child in for treatment and see improvement come back later to get help for themselves. Many popular men's health magazines and the media have helped to raise men's awareness of treatment for andropause, depression, and sexual dysfunction.

Andropause

Andropause is the decline of masculine hormones—in other words, the male form of menopause. Testosterone modulates the immune system, protects the skeletal system, and accounts for the characteristically "male" thought and behavioral patterns. In its absence, there is a gradual withdrawal of secondary sex characteristics, an increased incidence of osteoporosis, and perhaps an increased rate of infection/aging.

More than 25 percent of males over the age of sixty-five may have decreased testosterone levels; however, less than 5 percent of them are treated with hormone replacement. We have some ideas as to why hormone dysfunction in men is so often unrecognized and left untreated. First of all, much more is known about hormone transitions and replacement for women than is known for men. Most of the research on osteoporosis and hormone replacement has focused on menopause and women's health care concerns. Andropause has not been studied much at all. Second, women are accustomed to seeing a health care provider on a much more regular basis than men. Women usually see a physician or a nurse routinely for contraceptive measures, pregnancy, and other issues. They are used to talking to health care providers about changes in their bodies, emotions, and hormonal states and so find it natural to communicate menopausal or perimenopausal problems. Women notice changes early and go for help quickly. By contrast, a healthy man usually does not see a health care provider unless he is forced to by illness or injury. Because he doesn't require annual exams for birth control pills, PAP smears, and breast exams, he is unlikely to have established an ongoing dialogue with someone about hormonal transitions and problems. Oftentimes, men don't associate the emotional and physical changes they experience with hormone fluctuations, and if they do, they may not know who to talk to or how to talk about it.

The difficulty men have expressing themselves and getting their needs met when faced with major medical illness that has emotional impact is illustrated by a study reported in the September 2002 Oncology Nurses Forum. Large numbers of men with recurrent prostate disease reportedly experienced problems with side effects, anger, and pain. Men faced with this recurrent, serious disease experienced a negative impact on their leisure time and on their mental health. They had difficulty talking to health care professionals but at the same time expressed a need to talk to someone about their cancer. Many of them were unhappy with the information they received about their condition and the side effects of treatment. Clearly, in spite of wanting information and needing to talk to health care professionals about their emotional and physical problems, these men had trouble communicating and getting their needs met.

When testosterone levels decline, men experience emotional changes. Depression is the most common emotional problem men struggle with at this time in their lives. They have more daytime fatigue and feel run-down, and they frequently have disturbed sleep patterns. They feel irritable or restless and experience difficulty concentrating. They are moody and they have less self-esteem.

Physical changes also occur and men complain of weight gain or "spare tires around the middle" because muscle strength and density declines and is replaced by fat. Lifting power and physical endurance deteriorate. They notice their body hair is thinner. Illnesses may occur more frequently and injuries may not heal as quickly as before.

Loss of libido, or lack of sexual interest, is probably the most common concern among men who are experiencing hormonal imbalance problems. They may also experience impotence and testicular atrophy (testicles become smaller in the absence of testosterone).

RJ was fifty-seven years old when he first came for a psychiatric evaluation. He had seen his family doctor twice during the previous six months for vague complaints of "no energy, trouble sleeping, and feeling stressed-out." RJ's family doctor had determined that RJ was in good health and suggested an antidepressant for what sounded like a depressive illness. When RJ did not fully respond to two different antidepressants, he came to see us.

During the interview, RJ complained of characteristic signs of depression. He continued to struggle with irritability and sadness and sometimes felt mildly anxious; he was tired during the day and had trouble sleeping through the night. RJ didn't like feeling run-down with no energy to get through the day. He was extremely concerned about his decreasing sexual interest and occasional erectile dysfunction. He wondered if the antidepressants were to blame; so did we.

Because RJ was not experiencing improvement in his level of depression in spite of adequate doses of antidepressants, we suggested that his family doctor check some hormone levels, including thyroid function and testosterone. RJ's testosterone level was low and he was started on replacement therapy. During the next several weeks, his symptoms resolved.

Depression

Depression can be caused by testosterone decline, and the many conditions that men are at particularly high risk for compared to women can also precipitate depression in men. Head injuries, heart attacks, and strokes occur more commonly among males than females. The risk of having a depression remains elevated for as long as two years after one of these events. Men also take medications for heart conditions, parkinsonism, high blood pressure, and many other chronic medical conditions more frequently than women. Men who are experiencing symptoms of anxiety and depression need to have their medications reviewed for potential drug interactions and for the possibility that a medication is causing the symptoms or that one or more medications are preventing antidepressants from working.

Depression and anxiety disorders in men tend to be complicated by higher rates of suicide, substance abuse, and medical illnesses, and therefore the safety profiles of antidepressants are very important considerations. The SSRI medications are very safe for patients who have heart problems and for those who might impulsively take an overdose of medications. However, physicians need to educate men about the potential sexual side effects of the SSRI medications and the treatment for these complaints if they arise.

Sexual Dysfunction

Men are often very reluctant to bring up problems with their sexuality. They perceive any sexual difficulty as embarrassing and as a loss of manhood, so they are extremely uncomfortable discussing these issues. When we ask about sexual functioning, sexual problems, and side effects of treatment, we find that our male patients are relieved that we have opened the discussion and then willingly discuss their concerns. The sexual complaints that our male patients have typically fall into one of the following three categories: erectile dysfunction, premature ejaculation, and lack of sexual interest.

Erectile dysfunction is a man's failure to maintain an erection on a consistent basis. All men have failed to get or maintain an erection a few times in their lives (not that all of them will admit that in our experience) but this does not make a diagnosis of erectile dysfunction. The diagnosis is made when failure to maintain erections is happening often enough that a man's relationship is in trouble, and currently at least 25 percent of men over the age of sixty-five are affected. Some of the common causes of erectile dysfunction include treatment for prostate problems, high blood pressure, and diabetes, and medication side effects.

Surgery and radiation treatment for prostate cancer, diabetes, alcohol abuse, smoking, and high blood pressure can damage the nerves and blood vessels necessary for sexual response and functioning. Many medications can affect sexual functioning as well. Hormone therapy for advanced prostate cancer can cause erectile dysfunction.

Premature ejaculation (PE) is generally defined as a man's loss of erection either before intercourse or almost immediately upon penetration of his partner. Sometimes premature ejaculation is caused by anxiety or depression but very frequently the cause is unknown. In any case, there are several standard treatments. If a man has an untreated anxiety disorder or depression, he will benefit from treatment with an SSRI medication, especially Prozac or Zoloft. These medications have the side effect and, in this case, the side benefit, of prolonging the time it takes to reach a climax. If he does not have anxiety or depression, we still recommend the use of an SSRI since these have proved to be very effective interventions for PE. The SSRI medications may be effective for PE in lower doses than what is typically prescribed for depression and anxiety. Viagra is not generally used to treat this form of sexual dysfunction in men because it increases blood flow and sensitivity, thereby increasing the problem.

Lack of sexual interest has been discussed as a consequence of testosterone deficiency. It has a multitude of potential causes, including medication side effects, medical disorders, and psychiatric conditions. Many medical illnesses can cause men to experience a lack of sexual desire. Chronic pain conditions, neurological conditions such as seizure disorders or parkinsonism, and recurrent migraine headaches are examples of medical illnesses that inhibit sexual desire. Medications used to treat high blood pressure are widely prescribed and very often are a primary cause of sexual side effects.

Drug treatments for parkinsonism, ulcers, and psychiatric disorders all potentially decrease libido and many cause erectile dysfunction. Depression, anxiety, stress, and relationship conflict are also primary sources of decreased sexual desire in men.

Treatment

When a man is experiencing anxiety or depression, any underlying medical and/or neurological conditions must be identified and treated. Likewise, any medication or medication interaction that may be causing or aggravating symptoms of anxiety and depression needs to be identified and corrected. Next, substance abuse and lifestyle issues that are influencing the course of illness and that will interfere with treatment need to be addressed. This includes management of acting-out behaviors, diet, fitness, anger, and stress. Treatment of the primary anxiety and/or depressive disorder needs to be optimized with a prescription for health that often includes medication, therapies, dietary recommendations, supplements, fitness plans, relaxation training, and addressing spiritual needs. Men who are thinking about the addition of hormone replacement to their prescription for health should carefully consider the following information.

"Testosterone" scares some people. It makes them think of liver cancer and bodybuilders who abuse steroids, but that's not what we're talking about here. We're talking about physiological replacement—giving your body the amount it needs to restore it to the optimal level of functioning. If you were a diabetic, we wouldn't want you to take more insulin than you needed, and if you had a thyroid problem we wouldn't want you taking too much thyroid hormone replacement, either. The goal is to take the right amount for your needs. Doctors determine the amount of testosterone needed through blood tests. The type of blood test your doctor orders is very important. Some doctors like to order free testosterone levels. Others order total testosterone levels. To add to the confusion, laboratories have different levels that they consider normal ranges, but in general 300ng/dl is pushing the lower limit. Make sure your doctor orders a total testosterone level. The free testosterone level test is more expensive and you can determine your level of free testosterone from your total testosterone level test. Your free testosterone will be approximately 10 percent of your total testosterone. The other laboratory tests your doctor should order for you are prostate specific antigen (PSA), a complete blood count (CBC), and triglyceride and cholesterol levels. Testosterone can cause acceleration in the growth of prostate cancer, and therefore your doctor should also do a prostate check.

Testosterone is available in many forms—injection, oral, subcutaneous pellets, patches, gels—but most patients and doctors prefer the patches or gels. They are the easiest to use and are tolerated the best by most people. The patches are usually applied every twenty-four hours, and gel is applied daily. Testosterone is absorbed through the skin and avoids the liver. Dosing examples for testosterone replacement are: Androgel 2.5 to 5g applied daily or Androderm patch 2 to 2.5mg patch applied daily.

DHEA, dihydroepiandrosterone, is another hormone that is produced by the adrenal glands, and it, too, declines with age. DHEA is a precursor to testosterone, meaning it is converted to testosterone in the body. It has the same, although somewhat less potent, effects as testosterone on muscle strength, cognition, energy level, and so on. DHEA is an over-the-counter supplement that should be taken by men over the age of forty-five. The general dosing guidelines for DHEA are: 50mg daily for men over the age of forty-five, and 100mg daily for men over fifty-five.

All men should take vitamin C 500 to 1,000mg two to three times daily and vitamin E 400 IU twice daily. These are powerful antioxidants that offset the effects of aging and promote brain health and overall wellness. Vitamin E may be helpful in keeping oncogenes (genes that play a role in activating cancer) from turning on. Men should also take a multivitamin every day. Another very important daily supplement is low-dose (81mg) aspirin. Low-dose aspirin markedly reduces the risk of stroke and heart attack in men.

Growth hormone (GH) replacement is another very important topic to consider. Growth hormone is necessary for children to have normal growth and development but it remains important throughout life. Growth hormone production declines with age and usually decreases to 50 percent of its previous level by the time people reach their forties. It declines even further with advancing age. GH plays an important role in adulthood in muscle and connective tissue repair, maintaining muscle mass, regulating metabolic rate, building bone mass, and holding off many signs of aging. GH replacement therapy has been studied in the United States and elsewhere. The primary side effects of GH replacement in adults are fatigue and joint swelling. These side effects are minimized by starting replacement at low doses and increasing it gradually. Rarely, some men have developed increased breast size (gynecomastia), high blood sugar, or carpal tunnel syndrome while taking GH. Replacement levels are usually in the range of 0.03mg per kilogram of body weight injected subcutaneously (into the fat below the skin) three to five times weekly. When people use more than replacement amounts, they can develop what is called acromegaly. Think of a Neanderthal man and you'll get an idea of what you'll look like if you abuse GH. Your jaw and forehead will grow and enlarge, your skin will get thick and coarse, and the joints of your hands will get big.

Men should also have their thyroid function evaluated if they are experiencing fatigue, weight gain, increased need for sleep, or anxiety and depression that don't seem to be fully responding to treatment. Thyroid conditions commonly complicate the treatment of women, but they can affect men as well.

If you aren't on a fitness program, now is the time to start, and we can't stress this enough. Get on a high-protein diet and get rid of habits that don't promote your well-being.

CHAPTER 14

The Darkest Side of
Anxiety and Depression:
Suicide, Cutting, and Violence

Suicidal thoughts are common. One study reported that as many as 55 percent of the population have seriously considered suicide at some point in their lives. Unfortunately, suicidal behavior and completed suicides are also common. Often associated with untreated anxiety and depressive disorders, suicidal behavior often occurs when a person feels as though he or she has no other option in life. Suicide devastates a family, often leaving parents, spouses, and children feeling abandoned, guilt-stricken, and depressed. Women attempt suicide three times as often as men, yet men actually succeed in killing themselves three times more often than women. In general, the suicide attempts of women are less violent than the self-destructive acts of men. Women use drug overdoses, while men are prone to use hanging or guns. Women typically use suicide as a cry for help, while men typically hold back their feelings until they are overwhelmed and see no other option for healing their pain. Suicide is the eighth leading cause of death in the United States.

Brain SPECT studies have been useful in helping to further understand suicidal behavior. We have scanned more than 300 people who have attempted suicide. The majority of these patients had increased anterior cingulate activity (tendency to get stuck on negative thoughts); increased or decreased activity in the temporal lobes, most commonly on the left side (short fuse and irritability); and decreased activity in the prefrontal cortex during a concentration task (impulsivity and poor judgment). Most suicidal thoughts are brief in duration. Suicide is possible when someone gets locked into negative thoughts and has a short fuse and problems with impulsivity. Half of the suicides in America are committed when a person is intoxicated, because alcohol further suppresses prefrontal cortex function, taking the lid off of impulse control.

Another violent act toward one's self is cutting. In our experience, suicide and cutting often have the same underlying brain patterns as violence toward others. Suicide, cutting, and violence are complex human behaviors. There has long been a passionate debate over whether or not these behaviors are the result of psychological, social, or biological factors. Current research indicates that they are, in fact, the result of a combination of all these factors.

Due to the lack of specific biological studies to evaluate suicide, cutting, and violent behaviors, clinicians have had to rely on family history to look for genetic factors, along with a history of head trauma, seizures, or drug abuse to evaluate possible medical causes. One of the reasons underlying the lack of clear biological diagnostic tools may be the diversity and variability of the reported findings in the scientific literature. Nonspecific and conflicting EEG findings have been reported. A wide variety of neurotransmitter abnormalities have been reported, including disturbances of norepinephrine, dopamine, serotonin, acetylcholine, and gamma-aminobutyric acid (GABA). Numerous neuroanatomical sites have also been implicated in these behaviors, including the limbic system, temporal lobes, frontal lobe lesions, and prefrontal cortex.

Our SPECT studies provide a useful window into the brain of these patients and help bring together the diversity of biological findings. We have studied hundreds of children, teenagers, and adults who exhibited suicidal, cutting, and violent behavior and compared them to people who have never had these issues. Clearly, the brain patterns of these patients are different from those of the nonviolent person. We have found clinically and statistically significant differences between the suicidal and aggressive group and the non-suicidal and nonaggressive group. The results cluster around three major findings: decreased activity in the prefrontal cortex, increased anterior cingulate activity, and increased or decreased activity in the left temporal lobe. Other significant findings include increased focal activity in the left basal ganglia and on the left side of the limbic system.

The brain SPECT profile of these patients consists of one or more of the following:

- decreased activity in the prefrontal cortices (trouble with concentration and impulse control);

- increased anterior cingulate activity (getting locked into negative thoughts or behaviors; trouble seeing options);

- focal increased or decreased activity in the left temporal lobe (short fuse; dark, evil, awful, violent thoughts); and

- focal increased activity in the basal ganglia and/or limbic system (anxiety and moodiness).

It is very important to determine the nature and origin of these violent behaviors because that will predict appropriate treatment. For example, we often ask our patients to distinguish between impulsive (prefrontal cortex), compulsive (anterior cingulate gyrus), or explosive (left temporal lobe) aggression. Impulsive aggression happens on the spur of the moment, without forethought. Compulsive aggression occurs when someone cannot let a problem or hurt go. Explosive aggression is associated with dark, evil, violent thoughts and seems to come out of the blue for little or no reason.

JENNIFER

Jennifer, a thirty-two-year-old insurance agent, came to our clinic after trying to kill herself when a six-month relationship with her boyfriend ended. Jennifer's boyfriend had been attracted to her looks and intelligence but had become frustrated by her chronic lateness and her habit of picking fights for little or no reason at all. He felt stressed by the constant bickering and decided to terminate the relationship. Unfortunately he chose to announce his decision during dinner at a steakhouse in San Francisco, and Jennifer grabbed her steak knife and impulsively slashed her wrists. Crying, she said she didn't want to live anymore if they were not together. She bled all over the table, caused great turmoil in the restaurant, and was taken to San Francisco General Hospital. Jennifer calmed down while she was being cared for, felt embarrassed by her behavior, and promised not to do anything like that again. She was committed to a psychiatric hospital for three days and then released to our care. She came to see us because we had successfully treated her brother for ADD and depression.

As we got to know Jennifer, we understood her suicide attempt to be an impulsive act. She was motivated by her intense emotional upset, the immediate urge to escape her pain, and the need to inflict the same degree of pain on her boyfriend that she herself was experiencing at the moment. She had no true intention to kill herself and regretted the act as soon as she got to the hospital. Her SPECT scan showed decreased activity in her temporal lobes, especially on the left side, increased limbic activity, and decreased prefrontal cortex activity with concentration. With psychotherapy, an anticonvulsant to stabilize her temporal lobes, and a stimulating antidepressant (Wellbutrin) to calm limbic activity and enhance prefrontal cortex activity, she did much better—even better than before her suicide attempt.

Jennifer's Brain

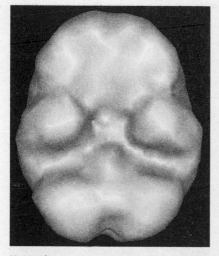 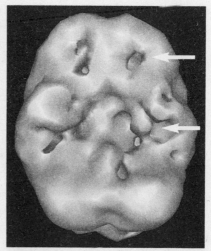

Normal
Underside surface view
Full, symmetrical activity.

Jennifer
Underside surface view
Decreased prefrontal cortex activity (top arrow) and decreased left temporal lobe activity (bottom arrow).

SHAWNA

Shawna, twenty-four, was referred to the clinic for persistent suicidal thoughts, cutting behavior, and temper problems. She had many scars on her arms, back, chest, and legs. A student at an East Coast university, she had tried many medications in the past that had not helped her. She said that she could not get away from the suicidal thoughts and that they were with her every hour of every day. The cutting, she said, helped to numb her emotional pain and distract her from the suicidal thoughts. She also had a flash temper that often ruined friendships and got her fired from a number of jobs. Shawna, like many people who cut or otherwise abuse themselves, had been sexually abused by her father and her brother. Her SPECT scan showed markedly increased activity in her anterior cingulate gyrus that caused her to get locked into negative thoughts and behaviors. Shawna's suicidal thoughts and cutting behaviors were very similar to obsessive-compulsive thoughts and behaviors. She also had markedly increased activity in her basal ganglia and limbic system and focal hot spots in her temporal lobes. These findings together are often seen in PTSD.

Shawna had a complex set of problem behaviors that required combination therapy. Medications were started to balance brain function. We have found that many cutters engage in this behavior to get an endorphin rush to help numb emotional pain. Endorphins are natural opiate, or morphine-like, substances in the brain that are released in response to pain or intense

Shawna's Brain

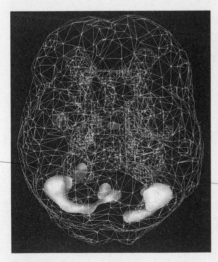

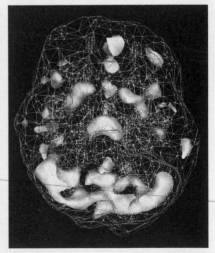

Normal
Underside active view
Good activity in the cerebellum; cool everywhere else.

Shawna
Underside active view
Increased basal ganglia, deep limbic, anterior cingulate gyrus, and deep temporal lobe activity.

exertion. Athletes have high levels of endorphins, which accounts for "runners' high" or the lift you experience after bodybuilding, mountain climbing, or extreme skiing. Pain also causes endorphins to be released, and some people cut themselves to release these natural painkillers in an effort to numb emotional pain. We put Shawna on Naltrexone, an opiate blocker. It stops the endorphin response and helps cutters stop cutting. On Naltrexone, cutting hurts. Shawna also needed an anticonvulsant and an SSRI to calm her temporal lobes and decrease the activity of her anterior cingulate gyrus.

Medication wasn't enough for Shawna. We believe medication is rarely enough for anyone and that "people need skills not just pills" for complete recovery. Because Shawna also had many symptoms of PTSD, we referred her for psychotherapy that involved EMDR (eye movement desensitization and reprocessing), a specific treatment for psychological trauma that has been found to help this brain pattern. With all of the treatments in place, Shawna was able to finish school and live without the intrusive suicidal thoughts, cutting, and temper problems.

Jim

When Jim, a twenty-nine-year-old fire protection engineer, was admitted to the hospital after separating from his wife of three years, he looked like a textbook case of depression. He was sad and tearful, and he had problems sleeping and couldn't concentrate. He thought about suicide and felt hopeless.

But Jim's depression had some of those "red flags" that make a good doctor want to spend a little more time sorting things out. For instance, he said he had a "very short fuse" and that during his marriage he and his wife had physically abused each other. In fact, Jim had spent time in the county jail for spousal abuse, and he abused people besides his wife. He yelled at other drivers on the road, and he was impatient with family members and inflexible at work. There were other worrisome symptoms such as brief periods of confusion, rage reactions in response to minimal provocation, and times during which Jim saw shadows out of the corners of his eyes. Jim's brain SPECT study revealed markedly decreased uptake in the deeper aspects of his left temporal lobe and decreased activity in his prefrontal cortex.

Jim had the clinical profile and SPECT findings that we know usually respond to anticonvulsant therapy. We also added a stimulating antidepressant. Although he continued to feel sad about the breakup of his marriage, he felt calmer and had better self-control, and his suicidal thoughts abated after he started on Tegretol and Wellbutrin. Jim later told us that he wished he had known about his brain dysfunction years earlier because he felt it might have changed the outcome of his marriage.

Violence Profile

Aggression is a complex process mediated by several different areas of the brain. Correlation of behavioral patterns to brain SPECT images of aggressive patients has enabled us to identify some of the areas involved in rage, violence, and self-destructive impulses.

We can say that in general the left hemisphere is especially involved in the genesis of violence. Decreased activity of the prefrontal cortex is one of the most commonly cited findings in people who have cognitive impairment (difficulty thinking clearly), as in schizophrenia or dementia. The prefrontal cortex is the organ of concentration, impulse control, and critical decision making. Violent offenders and aggressive people often misinterpret situations and react impulsively. Not surprisingly, they often have decreased activity of their prefrontal cortex.

Aggressive individuals may develop a pattern of obsessional thoughts in which they become "stuck" on real or imagined injustices and dwell on them. Examples of this type of thought process are men with road rage who, after being cut off in traffic, chase other drivers, and "jilted" lovers who develop stalking behaviors. Increased activity of the anterior cingulate gyrus is frequently present in this type of aggressive person. Studies have shown that medications that increase serotonin in the brain (such as Prozac or Anafranil) normalize activity in this part of the brain.

Increased activity in the basal ganglia is a SPECT finding that is often seen in patients with Panic Disorder or other anxiety disorders. Interestingly, many clinicians have reported a pattern of increasing anxiety in aggressive patients immediately prior to a violent episode. The violent patients report a sensation of mounting internal tension prior to lashing out at others.

Abnormalities in the limbic system have also been associated with aggressiveness. Some researchers discuss the concept of limbic seizures. Studies consistently find that when a structure called the amygdala, in the deep temporal lobes, often considered part of the limbic system, is stimulated, the person becomes more agitated and aggressive. The limbic system is often cited as the part of the brain that regulates mood. Abnormal activity in this area of the brain may be associated with significant moodiness.

Aggression associated with abnormalities in the temporal lobes has been described in numerous studies. This is perhaps the most striking finding of our work. Anticonvulsants such as Tegretol or Depakote are helpful in decreasing abnormal activity in this portion of the brain.

The temporal lobes can also be associated with fear, memory problems, aggression, and altered perceptions, such as illusions, frequent déjà vu, or hallucinations. In our experience, brain SPECT imaging is useful in identifying temporal lobe dysfunction. Traditionally, temporal lobe disorders have often gone unrecognized in psychiatry because these areas of abnormality are often found in the deep structures of the temporal lobes and are difficult to detect with routine EEGs. In fact, one study demonstrated that during active seizures, the EEG was positive in only 21 percent of cases. Brain SPECT, on the other hand, is a more sensitive tool than EEG for the diagnosis and localization of temporal lobe dysfunction.

In our experience with brain SPECT imaging, left-sided brain abnormalities are associated with patients who are more irritable and aggressive, whereas right-sided brain abnormalities more often correlate to patients who are more withdrawn, socially conscious, fearful, and much less aggressive.

ANDREW

In *Change Your Brain, Change Your Life,* Dr. Amen wrote about his nine-year-old nephew, Andrew, who attacked a little girl on the baseball field for no apparent reason. Eventually it was determined that he had a left temporal lobe cyst. At the time of the incident he appeared depressed, had aggressive outbursts, and complained to his mother of serious suicidal and homicidal thoughts (very abnormal for a nine-year-old). He drew pictures of himself hanging from a tree and shooting other children. When Andrew attacked the little girl on the baseball field for no apparent reason, his parents brought him to the Amen Clinic. As Dr. Amen sat with Andrew's parents and then with Andrew, he knew something wasn't right. He had never seen Andrew look so angry or sad. There were no explanations for Andrew's behavior. He did not report any form of abuse, other children were not bullying him, there was no family history of serious psychiatric illnesses, he had not sustained a recent head injury, and he had a wonderful family.

The vast majority of psychiatrists would have placed Andrew on some sort of medication and had him see a counselor for psychotherapy. Having performed more than 2,000 SPECT studies by that time, Dr. Amen wanted a picture of Andrew's brain before determining appropriate treatment. As Andrew's brain scan appeared on the computer screen, Dr. Amen thought a mistake had been made. There was *no* function in Andrew's left temporal lobe. It was determined that the scan was accurate, and while no left temporal lobe activity was a scary discovery, it was a relief to have an explanation for Andrew's aggressive behavior. The next day Andrew had an MRI (an anatomical brain study), which showed a cyst (a fluid-filled sac) about the size of a golf ball occupying the space where his left temporal lobe

Andrew's Missing Left Temporal Lobe
(3D underside surface view)

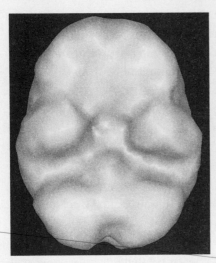 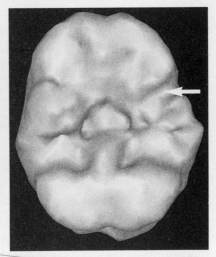

Normal
Underside surface view
Full, symmetrical activity.

Andrew
Underside surface view
Missing left temporal lobe (arrow).

should have been. We knew the cyst had to be removed. Getting someone to take this seriously, however, proved very frustrating.

Andrew's pediatrician was contacted and informed about the clinical situation and brain findings. The pediatrician contacted three pediatric neurologists about removing the cyst; all of them said that Andrew's negative behavior was probably not in any way related to the cyst in his brain and they would not recommend operating on him until he had real symptoms, such as seizures or speech problems. When the pediatrician reported back, Dr. Amen became furious. "Real symptoms!" he said. "I have a child with homicidal and suicidal thoughts who loses control over his behavior and attacks people." Dr. Amen contacted a couple of other pediatric neurosurgeons who had essentially the same response. While angry and appalled that the medical profession seemed unable to connect the brain to behavior, he wasn't going to wait until Andrew killed himself or someone else. Dr. Amen called the pediatric neurosurgeon Horhay Lazarette, M.D., at UCLA and told him about Andrew. He told Dr. Amen that he had operated on three other children with left temporal lobe cysts who were all aggressive and wondered at the commonality. Thankfully, after evaluating Andrew he agreed to remove the cyst.

When Andrew woke up after the surgery, he smiled at his mother. It was the first time in a year that he had smiled. His aggressive thoughts were gone and he reverted to the sweet child he used to be. It has not been an easy road for Andrew. Brain surgery is not without side effects. The cyst has refilled on a number of occasions. He had a shunt placed in his brain to drain the cyst, and altogether he has had thirteen operations.

In the summer of Andrew's fifteenth year, he became more irritable, unpredictable, and aggressive. Seemingly out of the blue, he took an overdose of prescription medication in a suicide attempt. Andrew was taken by ambulance to the emergency room. Fortunately, Andrew's vital signs were good and after he was medically stabilized he was taken to the adolescent psychiatric ward at UC Irvine. At the time, Andrew was rescanned. His left temporal lobe area was very abnormal (due to pressure from the cyst refilling) and he had a brain pattern we call the "ring of fire," which is diffuse hyperactivity of his whole brain. This pattern is often seen in patients who have cyclic mood disorders. Andrew had another brain surgery to alleviate the pressure near his left temporal lobe. In addition, he was placed on the anticonvulsant Neurontin 4,800mg and the antidepressant Effexor 225mg to stabilize and calm his brain. Over the next few months, Andrew's behavior normalized. His outbursts ceased, the dark thoughts were gone, and he was back to his sweet self. Yet he still struggled in school. Emotionally, he was doing so much better that Dr. Amen decided to order a follow-up scan to see his progress. The "hot" areas in the scan were significantly better. The

Andrew's Study Before and After Treatment

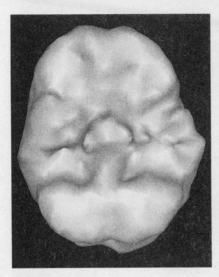

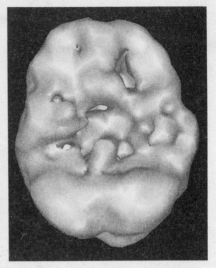

Before
Underside surface view
Missing left temporal lobe.

After
Underside surface view
Overall decreased activity in the
prefrontal and temporal lobes.

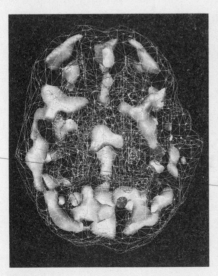

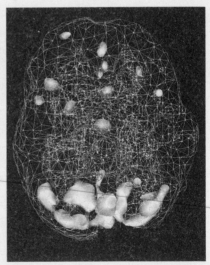

Before
Underside active view
"Ring of fire" pattern with
overall increased activity.

After
Underside active view
Overall calming of hyperactivity in the
brain.

"ring of fire" had been put out. But, in calming his brain, the medication had settled it down too much. Now his prefrontal cortex was much less active than before. Medications often do their job, but unfortunately they can also make some things worse. Seeing the lowered activity in the prefrontal cortex, Dr. Amen added a low dose of Concerta, a stimulant used to enhance prefrontal cortex function, to Andrew's regimen. Within two weeks Andrew had better energy, was able to focus, and did significantly better in school. The next report card was one of the best ones in his life. He has continued to excel in school with a balanced brain. He continues to be his sweet, loving self, when his brain works right.

CHAPTER 15

A Family Illness:
The Impact of Anxiety and
Depression on Families

nxiety and/or depression affect the whole family and often cause serious problems. We have seen "caring" families fall apart because of
the turmoil these illnesses generate. We have also seen divorces between people who "truly loved each other" because of the stress of one or
both partners having a mood or anxiety disorder. In addition, these illnesses
tend to have a strong genetic component, meaning if a parent has one type
of anxiety and/or depression, there is a high probability that one or more of
their children will have it as well. The stress that can break families apart
comes from many different sources.

Social isolation: Many people with anxiety and/or depression have struggled
in their relationships. To avoid experiencing pain again, they avoid relationships or make excuses to be by themselves. In addition, automatic negative
thoughts (ANTs) often cause them to put a negative spin on their past relationships so they are less likely to seek relationships in the future.

Misperceptions: Misperceptions often cause serious problems in relationships.
Often the parent or spouse of a person afflicted with anxiety or depression
has to spend an inordinate amount of time correcting misperceptions that
lead to disagreements. A patient's husband related the following story: One
night before he was leaving on a business trip, he told his wife that he was going to miss her. She thought he said, "I'm not going to miss you," and was
angry at him for the rest of the night, no matter what he said.

Lack of emotional expression: The partners of some people with anxiety and/or depression complain that there is little talking or emotional expression in the relationship. "He seems turned off when he comes home" is a common complaint.

Easily frustrated/emotional/moody: Many family members of anxious and/or depressed children, teens, and adults have told me that they never know what to expect from the person. "One minute she's happy, the next minute she's screaming" is a common complaint. Small amounts of stress may trigger huge explosions.

Tantrums/rage outbursts: Many people with anxiety and/or depression have rage outbursts, often with little provocation. After this occurs several times in a relationship, the parent, partner, or friend can become "gun-shy" and start to withdraw. Untreated anxiety and/or depression is often involved in abusive relationships.

Low self-esteem: When people do not feel good about themselves, it impairs their ability to relate to others. They have difficulty accepting compliments or getting outside of themselves to truly understand another person. The brain filters information coming in from the environment. When the brain's filter (self-esteem) is negative, people tend to see only the negative and ignore the positive. Many partners of these patients complain that when they give their partner a compliment, they find a way to make it look like they have just been criticized.

Chronic tension: People with anxiety and/or depression often feel restless and tense. This often causes them to search for ways to relax that may be inappropriate. They may use excessive sex, food, or alcohol to try to calm themselves. They also complain about excessive muscle tension and have frequent headaches, backaches, and sore joints.

Failure to see others' needs: Many people with anxiety and/or depression have trouble getting outside of themselves to see the emotional needs of others. They often appear spoiled, immature, and self-centered.

Low energy: Many people with anxiety and/or depression struggle with low energy levels. They often feel unable to engage in typical social activities and upset others who want to be with them or do things with them.

Lack of interest in usual activities or sex: Commonly, people with anxiety and/or depression experience anhedonia, or find little pleasure in things usually considered fun or pleasurable. They lose interest in sex, games, activities, and social contact. They tend to isolate themselves and avoid contact with others. Often, spouses take the lack of interest personally and feel very upset about the emotional and physical distance.

Lack of production: Lack of production is a also a common problem for families coping with anxiety and/or depression. A person with anxiety and/or depression may be unable or less able to work or do household chores. This puts an extra burden on other family members, who may feel resentment if they do not understand these illnesses.

When Untreated Brain Problems Interfere with Family Relationships

Underlying neurobiological problems can truly sabotage relationships.

- Deep limbic problems can cause a person to feel distant, disinterested in sex, irritable, unfocused, tired and negative.

- Basal ganglia problems cause sufferers to feel tense, uptight, physically ill, dependent, and conflict avoidant. Partners often misinterpret the anxiety or physical symptoms as complaining or whining and do not take seriously the level of suffering.

- Obsessive tendencies, as we have seen, cause rigid thinking styles, oppositional or argumentative behavior, holding onto grudges, and chronic stress in relationships.

- Prefrontal cortex issues, such as ADD, often sabotage relationships because of the sufferer's impulsive, restless, and distractible behaviors.

- Temporal lobe problems may be associated with frequent rage attacks, anger outbursts, mood swings, hearing things wrong, and low frustration tolerance.

Family Effectiveness Strategies

Families often fall victim to undiagnosed or untreated anxiety and/or depression. Involving the whole family in treatment is often essential for a healthy outcome. Get help early. Once you recognize the possibility that a brain problem is present, seek help. Often education is all that is needed to get people into treatment. The Amen Clinics have literally thousands of real-life stories of people who read one of our books and recognized their spouse, lover, parent, or child in a particular story and sought help. We have saved many relationships just by optimizing brain function.

Screen Other Family Members for Anxiety and/or Depression

Anxiety and/or depression usually have genetic underpinnings. When one member has one of these illnesses, it is more than likely that another person may have it as well. It is helpful to do some screening on every member of the immediate family. Trying to effectively treat a family when one or more members has an untreated case is an invitation to frustration and failure. We have found that when parents have untreated anxiety and/or depression, they have trouble following through on medication schedules for their children or the parent training suggestions given as part of therapy. When a sibling goes undiagnosed, he or she often sabotages the process by his or her own behavior.

Communication Issues

Families with one or more persons with anxiety and/or depression often have serious communication issues. There is a tendency to misinterpret information, react prematurely, or have emotional outbursts over real or imagined slights. It is essential to teach families how to listen, clarify misunderstandings, and avoid mind reading. It is also essential to teach families to communicate in a clear, unemotional manner. Emotionality decreases the effectiveness of communication.

Guilt

Guilt is an issue for many in families afflicted with a mood disorder. Resentment, bad feelings, and anger are common in family members, yet these emotions feel foreign and uncomfortable. Parents, spouses, and siblings feel that they are not "supposed" to have bad feelings toward people they love and are burdenened by feelings of guilt. It is essential to teach family members that these resentments are normal given the difficulties of the situation. Explaining the biological nature of these illnesses to family members often helps them understand the turmoil and be more compassionate toward the suffering person, while alleviating any guilt they might feel.

Split Families

Divorce is more common in families with anxiety and/or mood disorders. This may be due to many factors, such as increased family turmoil or substance abuse. Thus, the issues of divorce, custody, and stepfamilies often need to be addressed in treatment.

What to Do About Dad

Men are often the last people to admit that there are emotional or family problems. They often delay treatment, for their children or themselves, until there has been a negative effect on self-esteem or functioning. We have had many men tell us that there is nothing wrong with their son, even though he may have been expelled from school on numerous occasions three years in a row or is experiencing suicidal or aggressive behavior.

The reason men are less likely to see emotional or family problems is the subject of many debates. Here are some possibilities:

- many men have trouble verbalizing their feelings;

- many men have difficulty getting outside of themselves to see the needs of others;

- men tend to be more action-oriented than women, and they want to solve the problems themselves;

- societal expectations seem to be that men can handle problems on their own and they are weak if they seek help;

- men aren't allowed to cry or express any negative feelings, so they often do not learn to seek help or talk through their problems.

Whatever the reason, men in these families need education about anxiety and depression, and they need to be part of the treatment process for the best chance of success. To this end, it is important for wives, mothers, and therapists to engage fathers in a positive way and encourage them to see their valuable role in helping the whole family heal. Anxiety and mood disorders are family problems and need the support of everyone to be successful.

It is ineffective (and may be disastrous) to blame the man or make him feel like he is the cause of all the problems. Approach him in a positive way and he is more likely to be cooperative. Approach him in a negative way and there is likely to be resistance. In general, men are more competitive than women and need encouragement, as opposed to badgering, to be helpful. In our experience, once a resistant father becomes part of the treatment, he often takes much more responsibility for healing in the family.

While helping your partner get help, try to:

- have empathy for your partner and try to see the world through their eyes and the frustration and failure they have experienced;

- go to some appointments with the doctor together. When we treat adults with brain problems, we prefer to see both partners together, at least some of the time, to gather another perspective on the progress of treatment. We are often amazed at the different perspective we gain from a person's partner;

- get all the information you can. Both partners need clear education about the brain problem, its genetic roots, how it impacts couples, and its treatment;

- after the initial diagnosis, take a step back from the chronic turmoil that may have been present in the relationship. Look at your relationship from a new perspective and, if need be, try to start over;

- set up regular times for talking and checking in;

- set clear goals for each area of your life together and review them on a regular basis; evaluate whether your behavior is getting you what you want;

- set clear individual goals and share them with each other, then look for ways to help the other person reach their own personal goals;

- avoid stereotyped roles of "caretaker" and "sick one";

- talk out issues concerning sex, money, and child rearing in a kind and caring manner;

- frequently check in with each other during social gatherings to see the comfort level of each partner;

- get away alone together on a regular basis;

- work together parenting children. Children with brain problems put a tremendous strain on relationships. This is magnified further when one of the parents has a brain problem as well. See yourselves as partners, not adversaries;

- praise each other ten times more than you criticize;

- get rid of the smelly bucket of fish (hurts from the past) that you carry around. Many couples hold on to old hurts and use them to torture each other months or years later. These "smelly fish" are destructive and stink up a relationship. Clean them out of your life.

Gain Access to Your Own Good Brain

The internal conflicts associated with brain problems can ruin lives and families. It is essential to seek help when necessary. It is also critical for people not to be too proud to get help. Too many people feel they are somehow "less than others" if they seek help. We often tell patients that in our experience it is the successful people who seek help when they need it. Successful businesspeople hire the best possible outside consultants when they are faced with a problem that they cannot solve or when they need extra help. Unsuccessful people tend to deny they have problems, bury their heads, and blame others for their problems. If your attitude, behavior, thoughts, or feelings are sabotaging your chances for success in relationships, get help!

In thinking about getting help it is important to put these brain system problems in perspective. First, we have patients get rid of the concept of "normal versus not normal." There is no gold standard of "normal." We also tell our patients about a study published in 1994, sponsored by the National Institutes of Health, where researchers reported that 49 percent of the U.S. population suffer from a psychiatric illness at some point in their lives. Anxiety, substance abuse, and depression were the three most common illnesses. The same study reported that 29 percent of the population will have two separate, distinct psychiatric diagnoses and 17 percent will have three psychiatric diagnoses.

Most of us have traits of one or more brain system misfires. Sometimes the problems associated with each system are subclinical, which means they don't get in your way much, and sometimes the problems are severe enough that they significantly interfere with your day-to-day functioning. When they interfere, it is time to get help.

One of the most persuasive statements we give patients about seeking help is that we are often able to help them have *more access* to their own good brain. When their brain does not work efficiently, they are not efficient. When their brain works right, they can work right. We often show them brain SPECT studies to illustrate the difference in the scans on and off medication or targeted psychotherapy. As you can imagine, after looking at the images in this book, when you compare an underactive brain to one that is healthy, you want the one that is healthy.

What to Do When a Loved One Is in Denial About Needing Help

Unfortunately, the stigma associated with "psychiatric illness" prevents many people from getting help. People do not want to be seen as crazy, stupid, or defective and do not seek help until they (or their loved one) can no longer tolerate the pain. Men are especially affected by denial. Many teenagers also resist getting help even when faced with obvious problems. They worry about labels and do not want yet another adult judging their behavior.

Here are several suggestions to help people who are unwilling to get the help they need or are unaware that there is a problem:

1. Try the straightforward approach first (but with a new brain twist). Clearly tell the person what behaviors concern you. Tell them the problems may be due to underlying brain patterns that can be tuned up. Tell them help may be available—help not to cure a defect but rather to optimize how their brain functions. Tell them you know they are trying to do their best, but their behavior, thoughts, or feelings may be getting in the way of their success (at work, in relationships, or within themselves). Emphasize access, not defect.

2. Give them information. Books, videos, and articles on the subjects you are concerned about can be of tremendous help. Many people

come to see us because they read a book of ours, saw a video we produced, or read an article we wrote. Good information can be very persuasive, especially if presented in a positive, life-enhancing way.

3. When a person remains resistant to help, even after you have been straightforward and given them good information—plant seeds. Plant ideas about getting help and then water them regularly. Discuss relevant ideas, or pass along articles or other information about the topic from time to time. If you talk too much about getting help, people become resentful and resistant and won't seek help to spite you. Be careful not to go overboard.

4. Protect your relationship with the other person. People are more receptive to those they trust rather than those who nag and belittle them. Most people do not let anyone tell them something bad about themselves unless they trust the other person. Work on gaining the person's trust over the long run. It will make them more receptive to your suggestions. Do not make getting help the only thing you talk about. Make sure you are interested in their whole lives, not just their potential medical appointments.

5. Give them new hope. Many people with these problems have tried to get help and it did not work or it even made them worse. Educate them on new brain technology that helps professionals become more focused and more effective in treatment efforts.

6. There comes a time when you have to say enough is enough. If, over time, the other person refuses to get help and his or her behavior has a negative impact on your life, you may have to separate yourself. Staying in a toxic relationship is harmful to your health. Staying in a toxic relationship often enables the other person to remain sick. Threatening to leave is not the first approach to take, but after time it may be the best approach.

7. Realize you cannot force a person into treatment unless they are dangerous to themselves or others, or they are unable to care for themselves. You can only do what you can do. Fortunately, there is a lot more we can do today than even ten years ago.

CHAPTER 16

Help for Insomniacs

Many people with anxiety and depression also have insomnia. Sleep cycle problems disrupt energy cycles; interfere with performance at work, school, and in relationships; and compound the symptoms of anxiety and depression. Insomnia can prevent people from falling asleep (initial insomnia), disrupt sleep through frequent awakenings during the night (middle insomnia), and shorten the sleep cycle by causing early morning awakening (terminal insomnia). Sleep disorders can occur intermittently or transiently in response to stress, chronically or cyclically. These patterns are sometimes helpful in the diagnostic process. For instance, the symptom of sustained decreased sleep requirement in combination with elevated energy levels may indicate the presence of Bipolar (manic-depressive) Disorder. People who have terminal insomnia and morning fatigue with improved energy levels later in the day may have a form of major depression.

Some of the ways people with anxiety and depression have described their sleep problems are: "I have to count sheep to get to sleep, but the stupid sheep are always talking back to me"; "When I try to get to sleep all kinds of different thoughts come into my mind. It feels like my mind spins when I try to calm it down"; "The worries from the day go over and over in my head. I just can't shut my brain down"; "I have to sleep with a fan on to drown out my thoughts. I need noise to calm down."

Chronically disrupted sleep can wreak havoc in people's lives. For example, one teenager we know could hardly ever fall asleep before three o'clock in the morning. Consequently, he had trouble getting out of bed in the morning and was very tired during the day. Eventually he dropped out of school. Without adequate rest, his ability to learn and to form normal memory was impaired. School failure and dropping out of his peer group isolated him from other people his age. He went to the Stanford University

Sleep Center for help with his problem and in the end medication was needed to help normalize his sleep cycle.

Insomnia is one of the most common complaints in primary care practice. The number of adults in America affected may exceed 60 million, as reported in "Wake Up, America: A National Sleep Alert," National Commission on Sleep Disorders, Washington, D.C. 1993. Something that occurs so frequently should be easily diagnosed and treated but this is not the case. For one thing, the definition of "insomnia" can be elusive.

Patients have many different opinions about what constitutes insomnia, and many people who believe they are not sleeping enough are discovered to be sleeping more than the average person when evaluated by a sleep laboratory. Others who complain of insomnia don't realize that they are unintentionally doing something that disrupts their natural sleep cycle. For example, they may be drinking caffeine, eating sugar late in the day, drinking alcohol or smoking, taking naps during the day, exercising vigorously late in the evening, or staying up very late—all of which disrupt sleep cycles. Untreated medical and psychiatric illnesses and some medications disturb sleep, too.

The DSM-IV defines "insomnia" as a sleep disorder with complaints about the quality, duration, and timing of sleep. Sleep complaints must occur at least three times a week for at least one month and the patient must be impaired to some degree in his or her work, social, or school performance. Oftentimes people with insomnia have other problems, such as daytime fatigue, trouble concentrating, forgetfulness, depression, tension headaches, and difficulty with motivation, especially in the morning.

Insomnia interferes with people's quality of life. A self-administered questionnaire was given to 3,445 patients with one or more of five chronic major medical and psychiatric conditions who were recruited from the offices of clinicians practicing family medicine, internal medicine, endocrinology, cardiology, and psychiatry in three U.S. cities. Insomnia was independently associated with poor quality of life to almost the same extent as chronic conditions such as congestive heart failure and clinical depression. Insomnia aggravates other medical conditions such as CFS, fibromyalgia, and epilepsy. Insomniacs have more difficulty with job and academic performance because of fatigue and decreased concentration than people who do not suffer from insomnia. The cost of insomnia in terms of lost productivity and accidents has been estimated to be between $77 and $92 billion annually.

Sleep disturbance may be predictive of the onset or relapse of neuropsychiatric illness. Adults with sleep disorders have much higher rates of psychiatric disorders than the general population. They are at increased risk of developing subsequent anxiety disorders, depression, or substance abuse. The correlation between insomnia in survivors of motor vehicle accidents and the later onset of PTSD has been examined. The results show that patients who developed sleep complaints as early as one month after the motor vehicle accident later developed chronic PTSD and strongly suggest a predictive value for early onset insomnia in these trauma patients.

Sleep plays an important role in the formation of memory and normal learning activities. Think for a moment about how much more forgetful you are, how your concentration wanders, and how difficult it is for you to remember new information when you are tired compared to when you are well rested. Adequate rest and restorative sleep are vitally important to promote healing after brain injury from accidents or strokes, and yet the rate of sleep disturbance within the rehabilitation and traumatic brain injury (TBI) populations is very high. A study by the Rehabilitation Institute of Michigan found that only slightly more than half of TBI patients reported normal and satisfactory sleep and that complaints of difficulty initiating sleep were twice as common as problems with sleep duration among the TBI and rehabilitation populations.

Changes in biorhythms and disruptions of sleep cycles can trigger the onset of mania in bipolar patients. Sleep deprivation can also aggravate seizure conditions, and severe sleep deprivation can produce psychosis. Those of us who have worked in intensive care units (ICUs) are familiar with "ICU syndrome," a state in which a critically ill person becomes flooded by sensory input from all the lights, sounds, and activity going on around them. They are unable to sleep, or at least are deprived of REM (rapid eye movement sleep), for prolonged periods of time because of medication, interventions, and noise. Eventually they begin to hallucinate.

Generally, we see the less dramatic forms of insomnia. Insomnia that has troubled a person for less than a month is called acute or transient insomnia, and insomnia that is longer lasting is considered chronic insomnia.

Acute or transient insomnia is something that everyone has been bothered by on occasion. Some of the most common causes of transient insomnia are jet lag, minor stress or excitement, shift work, and trying to sleep in a new environment. This kind of acute insomnia usually goes away on its own or when the stressor is resolved. Herbal tea, self-relaxation, avoiding caffeine and alcohol, and exercise also help.

Chronic insomnia is more difficult to diagnose and treat. By far, the most common reason people develop chronic insomnia is another underlying condition that disturbs their sleep cycle. We call this type of chronic insomnia secondary insomnia. Doctors have to spend time trying to sort out whether or not a patient has secondary insomnia and, if so, what is causing it. The list of conditions that can cause insomnia is unbelievably long, so we have listed the most common:

- Medications—many medications including asthma medications, antihistamines, cough medicines, and anticonvulsants disturb sleep.

- Caffeine—coffee, tea, chocolate, and some herbal preparations contain caffeine and disrupt sleep.

- Alcohol, nicotine, and marijuana—although these compounds initially promote sleep for some people, they have the reverse effect as they wear off.

- Restless Legs Syndrome—a jerking motion of the legs or pedaling motion that drives a person's bed partner crazy (as well as the person who has it).

- Women's issues—pregnancy, PMS, menopause, perimenopause. During many of these hormonal transition times, a woman's sleep cycle may be disrupted every few minutes.

- Thyroid conditions.

- Congestive heart failure.

- Chronic pain conditions.

- Untreated or undertreated psychiatric conditions such as Obsessive-Compulsive Disorder, depression, and anxiety.

- Alzheimer's disease—dementia patients "sundown" or rev up at night and wander.

- Chronic gastrointestinal problems such as reflux.

- Men's issues—benign prostatic hypertrophy causes many trips to the bathroom at night, snoring, and sleep apnea (which are more common in men).

After all other reasons for insomnia have been ruled out or excluded, a patient can be diagnosed with primary insomnia. A doctor may also decide to send her patient to a sleep disorder laboratory for observation of their sleep cycle. Sleep labs are able to monitor patients with overnight polysomnography (PSG) and other tests that provide information about a patient's heart rate, breathing rate, oxygen levels, leg movements, brain waves, and eye movements during the sleep cycle. The results of these tests help make the diagnosis of sleep apnea, insomnia, and Restless Legs Syndrome.

Treatment

Acute or transient insomnia usually responds to the practice of good sleep habits (see How to Get a Good Night's Sleep, p. 280). We help our patients understand the effect of lifestyles, habits, and biorhythm fluctuations on their sleep cycle and how sleep requirements change depending on age. We help them identify stressors and problems that may be causing insomnia and recommend ways to manage them.

Sometimes, the practice of good sleep habits is not enough, as in the case of some shift workers who are unable to reset their sleep cycles on demand, or for people experiencing grief reactions who may suffer from insomnia for a few weeks to a few months during the acute grief phase. People who are hospitalized are another example of those for whom the practice of good sleep habits is not enough. In these and other cases, we prescribe medication on a short-term basis. Ambien and Sonata are two effective prescription medications currently available that are unrelated to the benzodiazepines (which can cause rebound insomnia, addiction, and withdrawal symptoms when discontinued). Ambien helps people fall asleep quickly and then wears off within seven to eight hours so that morning "hangover" effects or sedation are minimized. Sonata is a shorter-acting medication that lasts only about four hours and therefore can be taken either at bedtime to help trigger sleep or in the middle of the night by people who wake up and can't get back to sleep.

The benzodiazepines (BZPs) are traditionally used to treat insomnia and other sleep disturbances. There are many choices of benzodiazepines and they differ primarily in how quickly they take effect and how long they last. The ones that work for a long time, or have what we call a long half-life, are the ones that can cause morning sedation, or a hangover effect. Obviously, hangover effects are worsened if the medication is taken late at night, when it doesn't have enough time to wear off before the patient has to get up and start the day. BZPs work best for insomnia when they are used for short periods of time; otherwise, they lose effectiveness and cause rebound insomnia and withdrawal symptoms when discontinued. Alcohol should not be used by anyone who is taking a BZP because the central nervous system depressant action of the benzodiazepine class of drugs may be increased to toxic levels by alcohol. Other drugs that may interact in a potentially toxic way with BZPs are narcotic-containing painkillers, barbiturates, and some of the anti-anxiety agents, antidepressants, and anticonvulsants.

Desyrel (trazodone), an antidepressant, is not addictive and is unrelated to the benzodiazepines or to Ambien and Sonata. Since it is sedating it can be taken at night to help sleep on an as-needed or long-term basis. Anyone who is concerned about addiction or who cannot take the other medications described might try Desyrel. Desyrel can be taken along with most other medications; it has relatively few side effects other than sedation and does not cause significant rebound when discontinued. Men need to know that at higher doses Desyrel can cause priapism, painful sustained erections that require medical treatment. This is an uncommon occurrence but priapism is considered a medical emergency and any male taking this medication needs to be informed of the risk and told to immediately discontinue the drug and go to the emergency room if this rare side effect occurs.

Chronic insomnia requires a complex approach to treatment. Any underlying cause of chronic insomnia must be identified and treated. We must reiterate that chronic insomnia is most often caused by other underlying conditions and of these, depression, anxiety, substance abuse, psychological stress, and medication side effects are at the top of the list.

We begin treatment of chronic insomnia by educating our patients about sleep cycles, good sleep habits, things that influence sleep patterns, and the influence of age on sleep requirements. We help them set realistic expectations for sleep and treatment. Next we employ a treatment plan that incorporates the practice of good sleep habits (see How to Get a Good Night's Sleep, p. 280), treatment of any underlying condition, self-relaxation techniques, medication management, and cognitive behavioral therapy (CBT).

Patients who have difficulty getting to sleep frequently complain that thoughts keep them up at night. Sometimes they are anxious and therefore worry at night or obsess about problems. Other times, people say they feel fine but just can't turn off their mind and quit thinking. Nighttime thinkers need a form of CBT called imagery distraction. Imagery distraction is a technique in which an elaborate and interesting mental image or scenario is developed and focused on at bedtime in order to distract the insomniac from the other thoughts that keep them awake. Patients who practice this technique fall asleep more quickly and easily than those who don't. Biofeedback and self-relaxation techniques such as progressive relaxation, deep breathing, and meditation also decrease wakefulness and increase sleep time.

Medication management for chronic insomnia must be approached from the point of view that the patient may be taking medication intermittently or consistently for an extended period of time. This means that we generally do not prescribe medications from the BZP class because these drugs usually lose their effectiveness within six to twelve weeks. Patients would then need to increase the dose to be able to sleep and the pattern would repeat itself in a few weeks. Finally, when the medication no longer worked at higher dosages and was discontinued, the patient would experience rebound insomnia or withdrawal symptoms. Ambien and Sonata, on the other hand, can be prescribed for longer-term use. These medications have remained effective without dose adjustment for longer than a year, and patients have not experienced withdrawal or rebound insomnia upon discontinuation.

Desyrel is another option for patients who need long-term medication management and who do not derive benefit from Ambien or Sonata. It, too, can be used long-term. Other options are other sedating antidepressants or anticonvulsants, and we review these in the medication table that follows.

Naturopathic interventions may be helpful for either acute or chronic insomnia. Valerian root 450 to 900mg improves sleep for some people. It also has mild anxiety-reducing and muscle-relaxing effects. Valerian works through a different mechanism than benzodiazepines and the other medications. Results of several double-blind, placebo-controlled trials involving valerian for the treatment of insomnia showed that patients report improvement in the quality of their sleep and a decrease in the length of time it took for them to fall asleep when they used valerian. The benefits appeared to increase after several days of use. Higher doses of valerian were associated with reports of morning sedation. There are hundreds of different preparations of valerian available, and these preparations vary remarkably in the amount of volatile oils they contain. Pacific Rim sources may contain up to 8 percent volatile oil and some European sources as little as 0.5 percent. Bioavailability is a measure of how easily a compound can be broken down and metabolized by your body so that you can actually use it. To further confuse things, naturopathic compounds have an amazingly wide range of bioavailability and contaminants. Research your product if you want to use an herbal preparation. Visit *www.consumerlab.com* for additional information.

Sleep requirements change with age. Babies sleep a lot but unfortu-

Medications for Insomnia*				
Generic name	Brand name	Milligrams a day/ Available strengths	Times a day	Notes
triazolam hypnotic triazolo-benzodiazepine	Halcion	0.125 to 0.5/ 0.125, 0.25	bed-time	Short-acting benzo-diazepine that works quickly. Best for people who can't get to sleep. Can cause memory impairment, daytime sedation, and mild to severe with-drawal and rebound effects when abruptly discontinued. Abso-lutely no alcohol should be consumed while taking Halcion.
temazepam hypnotic benzodiaze-pine	Restoril	15 to 30/ 7.5, 15, 30	bed-time	Longer-acting than Halcion and therefore better for those who can get to sleep but can't stay asleep. Alco-hol should never be consumed with this or any other benzodi-azepine.
estazolam hypnotic triazolo-benzodiaze-pine	ProSom	0.5 to 2/ 1, 2	bed-time	Short-acting benzodi-azepine best used for short-term or inter-mittent insomnia. Frequently causes re-bound for the first few days after discontinua-tion. Alcohol should be strictly avoided.

Generic name	Brand name	Milligrams a day/ Available strengths	Times a day	Notes
zolpidem non-benzodiaze-pine hypnotic	Ambien	5 to 20/ 5, 10	bed-time	Can be used inter-mittently for acute insomnia or longer term. No associated rebound or withdrawal symptoms. Causes little hangover effect.
zaleplon non-benzodiaze-pine hypnotic	Sonata	10 to 20/ 5, 10	bed-time or as di-rected	Shorter-acting than Ambien and so can be used to treat night-time awakenings. Similar to Ambien in other ways.
doxepin TCA	Sinequan	10 to 300/ 10, 25, 50, 75, 100, 150	1 or 2 for depres-sion, or bed-time for in-somnia	Sedating TCA that can be used for insomnia in low to moderate dosages. Used in higher dosage for anxi-ety and depression.
imipramine TCA	Tofranil	10 to 300/ 10, 25, 50, 75, 100, 125, 150	1 to 2 for depres-sion, or bed-time for in-somnia	Also used for anxiety, panic disorder, bed-wetting, and depres-sion. May be used in low dosage for its sedating side effect to induce sleep.
mirtazapine antidepres-sant	Remeron	7.5 to 60/ 15, 30, 45	bed-time	Very sedating in low dose and can cause increased appetite as a side effect.

(continued)

Generic name	Brand name	Milligrams a day/ Available strengths	Times a day	Notes
trazodone antidepressant	Desyrel	50 to 400/ 50, 100, 150, and 150 divided tablet	bedtime, or divided doses for depression	This sedating antidepressant is frequently used for long-term treatment of insomnia. Not addictive, few side effects, no significant rebound when discontinued. Higher doses may cause priapism (painful sustained erections) in males.
gabapentin anticonvulsant	Neurontin	100 to 1,800+/ 100, 300, 400, 600, 800, and suspension	bedtime, or 3x/d for moodiness	Nontoxic anticonvulsant with wide dosage range that is sedating for some people at moderate to higher doses.
diphenhydramine antihistamine	Benadryl	25 to 100/ 25	bedtime	Available over the counter. Can cause moderate hangover effects at higher doses. No withdrawal symptoms and minimal rebound.
valerenic acids	Valerian root	450 to 900	bedtime	Naturopathic remedy that induces sleep and decreases nervousness for many people. Has mild muscle-relaxing properties. No rebound when discontinued. There are many preparations. Check *www. consumerlab.com* for help in finding a good brand.

*Note: There are many benzodiazepines, tricyclics, and over-the-counter compounds. This is only a representative list.

nately at the wrong time. Older adults usually require less sleep than they did as young adults, although this is sometimes hard to determine because older adults also nap more frequently than young adults. Teenagers require less sleep than babies but more than young adults. Their sleep cycle also seems to be shifted. They almost universally prefer going to bed later and sleeping later into the day than other age groups. Some middle to older teens go through phases during which they have increased sleep requirements. This is usually manifested by weekend sleeping marathons during which parents begin to wonder whether or not their teen is still breathing. A ringing telephone will rouse the teen and reassure parents.

Teenage insomnia is relatively rare and generally signals a serious issue such as Bipolar Disorder, severe depression, child abuse of some sort, or a medical condition. There is also a strong association between chemical dependence and sleep disorders in teenagers. Researchers at Henry Ford Hospital in Detroit, Michigan, are among those who have studied the link between adolescent substance abuse, sleep problems, and psychiatric disorders.

We believe that any child or teenager with a sleep disturbance should be carefully screened for the presence of medical and neurological causes. When these have been either eliminated or identified and treated, psychiatric causes should be considered. The most common psychiatric reasons for insomnia in the child and adolescent population are anxiety disorders, depression, Bipolar Disorder, psychotic disorders, abuse, and chemical dependence. Untreated psychiatric conditions in adolescence lead to increased rates of substance abuse. If your child or teenager has a sleep disorder, it may be a sign of something more serious.

Talking to Your Doctor

Collect and organize information about your sleeping pattern if you think you have a sleep disorder and you want to talk to your doctor about it. A simple journal or diary provides the best information and will give your doctor a clear picture of the type of insomnia or sleep disorder you have. Keep a record for two weeks of the time you go to bed, the number of minutes you think it took to fall asleep, how many times you woke up at night, what time you got up in the morning, and how many total hours you slept. Write down how long you nap each day. Make a note each morning about how rested you feel when you wake up. Make another note in the evening about how tired you are before lying down.

In addition to your two-week diary, you should give your doctor a list of all the medications you take and the time of day you take them. Don't forget to include herbal remedies, supplements, vitamins, and naturopathic interventions. Keep an estimate of how much caffeine, alcohol, nicotine, sugar, and starch you consume. If you have a bed partner, ask them to go with you to your appointment. Oftentimes your partner can provide a wealth of information about how restless you are at night and about breathing patterns, and these are important diagnostic clues. And, in the meantime, practice the good sleep skills below.

How to Get a Good Night's Sleep

- Get stimulants out of your system well before bedtime. If you take a stimulant for ADD or any other condition, try to take your last dose by early afternoon so it wears off before bedtime. Sometimes people with hyperactivity actually benefit from taking a stimulant before bedtime to calm them down so they can sleep. Stimulating antidepressants like Wellbutrin may need to be taken before 4 P.M. as well. Nicotine should be eliminated and caffeine should not be consumed for six to eight hours before bedtime. Caffeine is found in many things including tea, coffee, and chocolate.

- Don't take naps! This is one of the biggest mistakes people with insomnia make. They feel tired during the day, take naps, and compound their nighttime sleep-cycle disruption.

- Exercise during the day is very beneficial for insomnia, but it should be done more than four hours before bedtime. Vigorous exercise late in the evening often energizes people and keeps them awake.

- Alcohol, pain medication, and marijuana disrupt sleep. These compounds may cause initial drowsiness but as the body metabolizes them, they interrupt sleep. Avoid trying to fall asleep using these drugs.

- Plan for transition time. Almost everyone needs time to relax and unwind before going to sleep. Put aside busy or intense work and focus on calming activities before lying down.

- Don't use your bed for anything other than sexual activity or sleeping. If you can't sleep and are not engaged in sexual or sensual contact with your partner, get out of bed. Do not work, watch TV, read, write, or lie around awake.

- Move the clock. Clock-watching and trying too hard to go to sleep will cause more anxiety and aggravate your problem.

- Establish a regular sleeping schedule and stay on it even on the weekend. Changing sleep patterns by staying up too late or oversleeping on weekends is enough to trigger cycle disruptions in sensitive people.

- Pay attention to your environment. Your bedroom should be comfortable. Control the temperature and light.

- Reading might help you fall asleep but don't read anything too exciting, scary, or anxiety provoking. This applies to TV watching as well.

- A mixture of warm milk, a tablespoon of vanilla (not imitation vanilla, the real stuff), and a tablespoon of sugar can be very helpful. This increases serotonin in your brain and helps you sleep.

- If sugar makes you jittery or gives you an energy boost, or if you have ADD, avoid it beginning in the afternoon. You should avoid starches as well as they turn to sugar after you eat them.

- Sound therapy can induce a very peaceful mood and help relaxation. Some people like nature sounds; others prefer soft music, wind chimes, or even fans. Our clinic makes a sleep tape with a special sound machine that produces sound waves at the same frequency as a sleeping brain. The tape is played at bedtime and helps the brain "tune in" to a brain wave sleep state, which encourages a peaceful sleep.

- Sexual activity releases many natural hormones and muscle tension, and boosts people's sense of well-being. People with healthy sex lives usually sleep better.

- Meditation, massage, and warm baths are also very relaxing.

Sleep is critical. Use the techniques listed here to help. Be persistent. If one technique doesn't work for you, don't give up—try others.

CHAPTER 17

What to Do When
Treatment Doesn't Work

We have been able to help thousands of patients who were previously resistant to treatment through the new brain-based model outlined in this book. Although treatment failures are uncommon using this model, sometimes treatment doesn't seem to work or doesn't seem to alleviate a patient's symptoms completely. Patients who do not get well and those who get a little better but continue to experience significant symptoms in spite of what appears to be good treatment are known as "treatment-resistant patients." The most common reasons for treatment resistance can be grouped into six categories: problems with the diagnosis, medication issues, interfering factors, poor patient follow-through with treatment recommendations, trying to cut corners, and those things for which we do not have an explanation.

Problems with the Diagnosis

When a condition is misdiagnosed as anxiety or depression, treatment will be ineffective and often makes things worse by delaying treatment of the underlying illness. A classic example is thyroid illness. Hypothyroidism is a condition in which the thyroid gland is underactive. The decreased amount of thyroid hormone available to the body causes symptoms that mimic depression, such as fatigue, weight gain, changes in sleep pattern and appetite, decreased concentration, lack of motivation, and a downcast mood. This condition can easily be mistaken for depression and will not respond to antidepressant medication. On the other hand, an overactive thyroid gland can cause symptoms of anxiety, agitation, and increased heart rate that resemble anxiety disorders.

In our experience, ADD is one of the most frequently misdiagnosed conditions. ADD is a developmental disorder that presents early in life with symptoms of short attention span, distractibility, disorganization, procrastination, and impulse control issues. People with ADD often appear demoralized and are mistaken for people with depression.

Asperger's syndrome is another example of a condition that is easily confused with depression or anxiety. This autistic spectrum disorder is characterized by repetitive thoughts, rigid cognitive function, and very poor social skills. The internal distraction, academic difficulty, and preoccupation typical of this disorder cause Asperger's syndrome to be misdiagnosed as many things including depression, anxiety, and obsessive disorders.

The list of medical conditions that affect brain function and mood states is extensive and crosses all specialties from cardiology to dermatology. Medical conditions should always be excluded as the underlying cause of symptoms before a neuropsychiatric diagnosis is made.

Comorbidity is the presence of more than one condition and it is one of the more common reasons for poor treatment outcome. Substance abuse disorders are one of the most common comorbid conditions we treat. Marijuana, inhalants, pain medications, and alcohol abuse interfere with the action of prescription medications used to treat anxiety and depression. Substance abuse disturbs brain function and can disrupt brain development. Almost everyone knows this is true for babies exposed to substances during development, but most people don't realize that teenagers and young adults are still vulnerable because their brains are still developing into young adulthood.

Self-medication with drugs and alcohol is a vicious cycle. Emotional and physical pain cause people to abuse substances or misuse prescription medications in an attempt to get relief, but intoxication and withdrawal states only aggravate the underlying conditions. Substance abuse issues must be dealt with for treatment to be effective.

Finally, doctors do not always get all the information necessary to make a correct diagnosis or to make treatment decisions. Sometimes patients do not tell us about underlying medical conditions, substance abuse, other medications they are taking, or the amount of stress in their lives. The reasons people withhold information are as unique as the people themselves. Many times people feel shame over things in their past; think we won't treat them if they have a substance abuse problem; are embarrassed by their thoughts; believe they will be judged if they reveal they are HIV positive; are concerned about what will be written in the medical record; and so on.

Other times people forget about a prior head injury or cannot remember the names and dosages of the medications they are taking. We can tell you with absolute certainty that all of this information is vitally important for the accurate rendering of a diagnosis and formation of an effective treatment plan. Physicians would much rather have their patients bring up a concern and discuss how the information will be protected than jeopardize the diagnosis and treatment plan.

Medication Issues

Think of your treatment plan as a recipe and your medication as one of the ingredients in the recipe. If you leave things out or make additions or substitutions, or if your timing is off, you may not get what you planned for. But if you follow the recipe, you will have a better product. Medications work best when they are taken on schedule. They work less well if they are taken randomly, and they don't work at all when doses are missed frequently. Why do people miss doses of medication? Complicated dosing schedules are sometimes a problem and this is the reason we try to use medications that can be taken once or twice daily. We also try to minimize the number of medications a person is taking to further simplify things. The very young, very old, and people with ADD may not remember to take all their doses. Teenagers sometimes skip doses intentionally, and unfortunately some parents who are in divorced or separated situations victimize their children by withholding medication to get back at the other parent.

Medication must be taken at the correct dose to be effective. Every day in our practice we are amazed by the number of treatment-resistant patients who are simply underdosed on their medications. Taking only half of the Prozac or Neurontin necessary to help your brain will not work any better than using half the heat necessary to bake your bread. Additionally, many doctors who are not specialists in the field of psychiatry do not prescribe high enough doses of neurological and psychiatric medications.

Other prescription medications, over-the-counter drugs, and herbs and supplements can interfere with the action of medications prescribed to treat anxiety and depression. Examples of medications that may cause such interference include some of the antihistamines, asthma medications, and medications used to treat heart conditions. Caffeine is known to aggravate some of the antidepressant side effects. Medications used to treat high blood pressure cross over into brain tissue and worsen depression. Kava kava, an herbal supplement, was recently withdrawn from the European market because it has been implicated in liver failure, and St. John's wort can interact with several antidepressants. It is extremely important always to inform all your doctors of every medication and supplement you take.

We have also seen generic medications cause treatment problems and confusion, and we know generic medication works differently from brand-name medication. Sometimes it works better, sometimes worse. For example, a close friend of ours with Pure Anxiety responds very nicely to a specific generic form of imipramine. She does not respond at all to brand-name imipramine (Tofranil).

One factor that few physicians consider is the difference between how females and males process medication. Very few drug trials involve women and therefore finding the therapeutic dose for women is often a process of trial and error. Hormonal factors affect the action of medications in women. Many women also have a higher percentage of body fat than men and that may affect drug distribution. These and other factors mean that women may need a different dose of the same medication we use to treat men or else an altogether entirely different protocol.

Interfering Factors

Your treatment plan is a prescription for health, and when prescribed lifestyle changes are not made the entire plan can be sabotaged. We prescribe dietary changes to help brain function, boost medication effectiveness, and normalize energy levels, as part of an overall health plan. Patients eating a high-carbohydrate diet will continue to experience blood sugar and insulin-level fluctuations that aggravate their moods, energy levels, and ability to concentrate. Excessive caffeine and any nicotine use will interfere with the action of many medications, including stimulants. Because the effects of caffeine and nicotine are so short-lived, they cause people to be irritable and sometimes more depressed. They decrease blood flow and deprive the brain of oxygen. Citrus juices slow down the ability of the body to process some medications.

Exercise is one of the most overlooked and underused interventions. Aerobic exercise boosts the body's immune system, increases oxygen delivery to the brain, and increases the release of endorphins, neurotransmitters in the brain that promote a sense of well-being. Exercise is a wonderful stress-management technique.

Stress is not the enemy. The word is so overused these days that some of us consider it almost meaningless. In fact, events that most of us would welcome in our lives—financial gain, a move into a new home, the birth of our first child, and so on—produce the same physiological changes as the events most of us wish we could avoid in our lives, like the death of a family member. It isn't the happy or sad events that happen in life that are the problem; rather, the problem is our occasional lack of effectiveness in coping with them. The failure of healthy coping mechanisms interferes with treatment and causes an excessive release of corticosteroids from the adrenal glands. These stress hormones circulate to the brain, damaging cells, especially in the temporal lobes. Failure of coping mechanisms must be treated with the appropriate therapy to maximize outcome.

A problematic or difficult environment (such as at home, work, or school) also contributes to treatment failure. You can have the right diagnosis and right treatment protocol, but if you are in a chronically difficult marriage, have difficult parents or teachers, or have siblings who are abusing you, treatment will appear flawed and frequently fail. The environment needs to support the treatment.

One of the most important aspects of the treatment plan is the therapeutic relationship. The doctor-patient relationship is in itself an instrument of healing. Patients work hard to find care providers who are not only experts in their field but who also are good communicators. Conflicts and miscommunication in doctor-patient or patient-therapist relationships lead to poor outcomes. Patients need to inform all medical providers of any change in their medical or psychological status and report any medications, supplements, herbs, and over-the-counter medications they are taking.

Poor Patient Follow-through

Lack of patient follow-through with treatment is what doctors and therapists call "lack of compliance." Doctors spend a lot of time trying to figure out why patients become noncompliant with treatment protocols. We've compiled our own list of common reasons:

- Patients expect medications to work too quickly and discontinue their use before the medications have a chance to be effective.

- Doctors, especially those who are not specialists in neuropsychiatry, change patient medications prematurely or do not push doses high enough for the medications to be effective. Patients need to see specialists for treatment of their disorders.

- Medication dosing schedules are complicated or multiple medications are prescribed and patients become frustrated.

- Side effects occur, and sometimes patients are not told to expect them, and/or the doctor does not know how to treat the side effects.

- Patients stop medications as soon as they start to feel better and then relapse.

- Well-meaning family members and friends undermine the treatment plan by reassuring patients that they "don't really need medicine" and suggesting alternatives such as meditation, exercise, and religion. We believe these are essential elements of a treatment plan but alone they absolutely will not treat anxiety and depression.

- Popular media and the Internet are rife with sensational stories and hype that scare patients into prematurely discontinuing their treatment.

- Sometimes patients expect too much from medications. There are no magic bullets and medications are only one part of a prescription for health.

- Patients are not willing to discontinue the use of drugs and/or alcohol, participate in therapy, or make other lifestyle changes that are necessary to achieve the best outcomes.

To increase the likelihood that our patients will derive the best possible benefit from treatment, we stress the importance of strict compliance with the full treatment plan. A full treatment plan is a prescription for health that encompasses many areas of your life and requires your active participation on a daily basis. Communication with your doctor about your concerns and to modify the plan as needed is essential. Patience and persistence are keys to success.

Impatience and thoughtlessness can have dire consequences. Dr. Amen had a patient with Overfocused Anxiety/Depression who responded very nicely to a combination of medication and dietary changes. After two years of benefit this patient stopped her medication because someone at her church told her there was negative information in Internet chat rooms about her medication. Within a few weeks, she was as symptomatic as before, and when she resumed her medication it did not work as well. It took us almost eighteen months to help her feel more balanced. It is not unusual for medications that were previously working beautifully to be less effective when patients discontinue them prematurely and then resume taking them.

Cutting Corners

We've all heard the phrase "You get what you pay for." Unfortunately, we usually hear it after we've written a check for something we were sure was a good bargain, only to realize we have a "lemon" on our hands the day after the warranty runs out. No one wants to spend money needlessly and everyone wants to make a good investment. We believe the best investment you can make is in your health, especially your brain health. This truly is an investment for life—your own life and the lives of your children.

Most of us complain less about the cost of the clothing, food, and automobiles than we do about the health care we purchase. Many of us spend money excessively on entertainment, large homes, vacations, and even things that are not good for us, such as cigarettes, excessive alcohol, and too much food. These things are all expensive, and so is health care.

Some patients are treated by non-specialists and do fine on generic drugs. But if you are among those who are becoming frustrated because you are not getting better, you need to see a specialist. You might benefit from technology that can image your brain and guide diagnosis and treatment. You might need a more sophisticated combination of medications or brand-name medications. This might require some people to pay out of pocket or go outside their insurance plan. The cost of a consultation with a specialist, with or without tests, and getting the correct treatment prescribed is enormously less expensive than the costs of repeated visits to other doctors, medication trials and errors, and long-term disability from poorly treated symptoms.

The Unknown

In almost every psychiatrist's practice, almost one-third of depressed patients can be classified as chronically depressed. Major Depressive Episode with incomplete interepisode remission, double depression, Dysthymia, and chronic major depression are the types of chronic depressive disorders found in the DSM-IV. Poor compliance, premature discontinuation of treatment, active substance abuse, and untreated medical illnesses are some of the factors that contribute to the risk of continued symptoms of depression and anxiety. Untreated sleep disturbances are known to increase the risk of chronic anxiety and depression.

We think of every patient as having a chance of relapse or recurrence because we know that depression and anxiety are much more likely than not to come back at some point. The risk of relapse is much higher for patients who are treated only until their symptoms respond as opposed to those who are treated until their symptoms are in remission. In other words, patients who discontinue medications on their own or on their doctor's advice as soon as they start to feel better are at much higher relapse risk than those who remain on medication until they complete a full course (usually several years). Further, once in remission, the chance of relapse and recurrence can be further reduced by maintenance therapy.

In studies where patients are randomly assigned to antidepressant therapy versus placebo for maintenance therapy and followed for more than two years, patients on antidepressants had lower rates of relapse and the relapse risk was greatest within the first six months. All patients should know that maintenance therapy is an option for them and it often helps prevent further episodes.

Maintenance therapy is the long-term administration of medication at full dose or at the highest dose necessary to control symptoms. Any patient who has had more than one episode of illness, one particularly difficult episode, or an episode with complicating factors such as psychosis or suicidal thoughts; who has a cyclic pattern of illness; or who just can't have their lives derailed by illness should be on maintenance therapy.

There are countless factors that influence the neurochemical state of the mind and body. We are only just beginning to understand some of these influences and there is much we do not know. We look forward to the continued development of imaging techniques to study the brain, to guide treatment, and to follow the course of treatment. New drugs and drug delivery systems are improving treatment response while limiting side effects. Surgical techniques are being refined that may soon offer patients permanent relief from symptoms without the need for drug therapy.

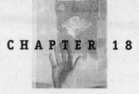

CHAPTER 18

How to Find the Help You Need:
A Resource Guide

Four questions we are frequently asked are: When is it time to see a professional about anxiety or depression? What do I do when a loved one is in denial about needing help? How do I go about finding a competent professional? When do you order a SPECT study? These questions are answered in this chapter in detail. We also provide a comprehensive referral list of physicians and therapists throughout the country who use our brain-based model.

When Is It Time to See a Professional About Anxiety or Depression?

This question is relatively easy to answer. We recommend people seek professional help for themselves or a family member when their behaviors, feelings, or thoughts interfere with their ability to reach their potential in their relationships, work, or academically. If you are experiencing persistent relationship struggles (parent-child, with siblings or friends, romantic), it's time to get help. If you have ongoing school or work problems related to anxiety or depression, it is time to get professional help. If your impulsive behavior or poor choices are causing consistent monetary problems, it's time to get help. Many people have told us they cannot afford to get professional help. We respond that it is much more costly to live with untreated anxiety or depression than it is to get appropriate help.

As discussed previously, pride can get in the way of seeking a proper diagnosis. People want to be strong and self-reliant. We are constantly reminded of the strength it takes to make the decision to get help. Also, getting help should be looked at as a way to get your brain operating at its full capacity.

Jeff was the twenty-two-year-old son of an attorney. His mother brought him to see us because he had problems in school and he was moody. He was angry, resentful, and oppositional, and his mood was unpredictable. He had been in psychotherapy with a number of different therapists over the past twelve years. His mother thought that medication might be helpful. Jeff was opposed. "I don't want to be on medication," he almost shouted. "I want to be myself." His SPECT study revealed markedly decreased temporal lobe activity, increased anterior cingulate gyrus activity, and decreased prefrontal cortex activity. Dr. Amen showed him his brain scan on the computer monitor. After he understood the scan, his first question was, "Can you give me something to help my brain?" He was given medication to stabilize his temporal lobe and supplements to calm his anterior cingulate gyrus and stimulate his prefrontal cortex. He felt better within several weeks. Jeff was compliant with treatment because he wanted to have optimal access to his own brain.

What to Do When a Loved One Is in Denial About Needing Help

Many men, when faced with obvious problems in their marriage, with their children, or even in themselves, refuse to see problems. Their lack of awareness and strong tendency toward denial prevent them from seeking help until more damage than necessary has been done. Many men have to be threatened with divorce before they seek help. Some people may say it is unfair of us to pick on men. And, indeed, some men see problems long before some women. Overall, however, mothers see problems in children before fathers and are more willing to seek help, and many more wives call for marital counseling than husbands. What is it in our society that causes men to overlook obvious problems, to deny problems until it is too late to deal with them effectively or until more damage is done than necessary? Some of the answers may be found in how boys are raised in our society, the societal expectations we place on men, the overwhelming pace of many men's daily lives, and the brain.

Boys most often engage in active play (sports, war games, video games, etc.) that involves little dialogue or communication. The games often involve dominance and submissiveness, winning and losing, and little interpersonal communication. Force, strength, and skill handle problems. Girls, on the other hand, often engage in more interpersonal or communicative types of play, such as dolls and storytelling. Fathers often take their sons out to throw the ball around or shoot hoops, rather than go for a walk and talk.

Many men retain the childhood notions of competition and that one must be better than others to be any good at all. To admit to a problem is to be less than other men. As a result, many men wait to seek help until their problem is obvious to the whole world. Other men feel totally responsible for all that happens in their families and admitting to a problem is admitting that they have in some way failed.

Clearly, the pace of life prevents some men from being able to take the time to look clearly at the important people in their lives and their relationships with them. When we spend time with fathers and husbands and help them slow down enough to see what is really important to them, more often than not they begin to see the problems and work toward more helpful solutions. The issue is not one of being uncaring or uninterested; it is not seeing what is there.

Men are wired differently than women. Men tend to be more left-brained, which gives them better access to logical, detail-oriented thought patterns. Women tend to have greater access to both sides of their brains, with the right side being involved in understanding the gestalt, or big picture, of a situation. The right side of the brain seems to be involved in being able to admit to a problem. Many men just don't see the problems with anxiety or depression even though the symptoms may be very clear to others.

For several suggestions to help people who are in denial about needing help, please refer to pages 267–268.

Finding a Competent Professional Who Uses This New Brain Science Thinking

We get an estimated forty to fifty calls, faxes, or e-mails a week from people all over the world looking for competent professionals in their area who think in similar ways to the principles outlined in this book. Because this approach is on the edge of what is new in brain science, other professionals may be hard to find. However, finding the right professional for evaluation and treatment is critical to the healing process. The right professional can have a very positive impact on your life. The wrong professional can make things worse. There are a number of steps to take in finding the best person to assist you.

1. Get the best person you can find. Saving money up front may cost you in the long run. The right help is not only cost effective but saves unnecessary pain and suffering. Don't rely only on a person in your managed care plan. That person may or may not be a good fit for you. Search for the best. If he or she is in your insurance plan—great. Don't let that be the primary criterion.

2. Use a specialist. Diagnosis and treatment for anxiety and depression are expanding at a rapid pace. Specialists keep up with the details in their fields, while generalists (family physicians) have to try to keep up with everything. If you have a heart arrhythmia, you would see a cardiologist rather than a general internist. You want someone to treat you who has seen hundreds or even thousands of cases like yours.

3. Once you get the names of competent professionals, check their credentials. Very few patients ever check a professional's background. Board certification is a positive credential. To become board certified, physicians have to pass additional written and verbal tests. They have had to discipline themselves to gain the skill and knowledge that were acceptable to their colleagues. Don't give too much weight to the medical school or graduate school the professional attended. We have worked with some doctors who went to Yale and Harvard who did not have a clue about how to treat patients appropriately, while other doctors from less prestigious schools were outstanding, forward-thinking, and caring.

4. Set up an interview with the professional to see whether or not you want to work with him or her. Generally you have to pay for their time, but it is worth spending time getting to know the people you will rely on for help.

5. Read the work of the professional or hear him or her speak, if possible. Many professionals write articles or books or speak at meetings or local groups. By doing so you may be able to get a feel for the kind of person they are and their ability to help you.

6. Look for a person who is open-minded, up to date, and willing to try new things.

7. Look for a person who treats you with respect and who listens to your questions and responds to your needs. Look for a relationship that is collaborative and respectful.

We know it is hard to find a professional who meets all of these criteria who also has the right training in brain physiology, but these people can be found. Be persistent. The caregiver is essential to healing.

Frequently Asked Questions About SPECT

Here are several common questions and answers about SPECT.

Will the SPECT study give me an accurate diagnosis? No. A SPECT study by itself will not give a diagnosis. SPECT studies help the clinician understand more about the specific function of your brain. Each person's brain is unique, which may lead to unique responses to medicine or therapy. Diagnoses about specific conditions are made through a combination of clinical history, personal interview, information from families, diagnostic checklists, SPECT studies, and other neuropsychological tests. No study is "a doctor in a box" that can give accurate diagnoses on individual patients.

Why are SPECT studies ordered? Some common reasons include:

1. evaluating seizure activity;

2. evaluating blood vessel diseases, such as stroke;

3. evaluating dementia and distinguishing between dementia and pseudodementia (depression that looks like dementia);

4. evaluating the effects of mild, moderate, and severe head trauma;

5. suspicion of underlying organic brain condition, such as seizure activity contributing to behavioral disturbance, prenatal trauma, or exposure to toxins;

6. evaluating atypical or unresponsive aggressive behavior;

7. determining extent of brain impairment caused by drug or alcohol abuse;

8. typing anxiety, depression, and attention deficit disorders when clinical presentation is not clear.

Do I need to be off medications before the study? This question must be answered individually between you and your doctor. In general, it is better to be off medications until they are out of your system, but this is not always practical or advisable. If the study is done while on medications, let the technician know so that when the physician reads the study he will include that information in the interpretation of the scan. In general, we recommend patients try to be off stimulants for at least four days before the first scan and remain off them until after the second scan, if one is ordered. It is generally not practical to stop medications such as Prozac because they last in the body for four to six weeks. Check with your specific doctor for recommendations.

What should I do the day of the scan? On the day of the scan, decrease or eliminate your caffeine intake and try not to take cold medication or aspirin (if you do, please make a note of it on the intake form). Eat as you normally would.

Are there any side effects or risks to the study? The study does not involve a dye and people do not have allergic reactions to the study. The possibility exists, although in a very small percentage of patients, of a mild rash, facial redness and edema, fever, and a transient increase in blood pressure. The amount of radiation exposure from one brain SPECT study is approximately the same as one abdominal X ray.

How is the SPECT procedure done? The patient is placed in a quiet room and a small intravenous (IV) line is started. The patient remains quiet for approximately ten minutes with his or her eyes open to allow their mental state to equilibrate to the environment. The imaging agent is then injected through the IV. After another short period of time, the patient lies on a table and the SPECT camera rotates around his or her head (the patient does not go into a tube). The time on the table is approximately fifteen minutes. If a concentration study is ordered, the patient returns on another day.

Are there alternatives to having a SPECT study? In our opinion, SPECT is the most clinically useful study of brain function. There are other studies, such as electroencephalograms (EEGs), positron emission tomography (PET) studies, and functional MRIs (fMRI). PET studies and fMRI are considerably more costly and are performed mostly in research settings. EEGs, in our opinion, do not provide enough information about the deep structures of the brain to be as helpful as SPECT studies.

Does insurance cover the cost of SPECT studies? Reimbursement by insurance companies varies according to your plan. It is often a good idea to check with your insurance company ahead of time to see if it is a covered benefit.

Is the use of brain SPECT imaging accepted in the medical community? Brain SPECT studies are widely recognized as an effective tool for evaluating brain function in seizures, strokes, dementia, and head trauma. There are literally hundreds of research articles on these topics. In our clinic, based on our experience for more than a decade, we have developed this technology further to evaluate aggression and nonresponsive psychiatric conditions. Unfortunately, many physicians do not fully understand the application of SPECT imaging and may tell you that the technology is experimental, but more than 350 physicians in the United States have referred patients to us for scans.

Referral Resources

There are not centers like ours around the country. But there are many forward-thinking physicians and psychotherapists who understand the connection between the brain and behavior. Here is a list of professionals across the country to whom we refer.

Physicians

Alabama

John Bailey, M.D.
829 S. University Blvd.
Mobile, AL 36609
251/342-6443
Board-certified family physician; practice limited to adult and child ADHD, LD, depression, and Bipolar Disorder.

Arizona

Eric Greenman, M.D.
932 West Chandler Blvd.
Chandler, AZ 85225
480/786-9000, fax 480/786-5190
Child, adolescent, adult psychiatry.

California

Los Angeles Area

Leonard (Skip) Baker, M.D.
USC Clinical Professor of Pediatrics
Descanso Medical Center for Development and Learning
1346 Foothill Blvd., #301
La Canada, CA 91011
818/790-1587, fax 818/952-3473
Behavioral pediatrics.

Thomas Brod, M.D.
12304 Santa Monica Blvd., #210
Los Angeles, CA 90025
310/207-3337
Older adolescent and adult psychiatry.

Hyla Cass, M.D.
1608 Michael Lane
Pacific Palisades, CA 90272
310/459-9866
www.cassmd.com
Expert in natural treatments.

Steven Lawrence, M.D.
3424 Carson St., #580
Torrance, CA 90503
310/542-7878, fax 310/542-9858
Child, adolescent, and adult psychiatry.

Jack H. Lindheimer, M.D.
4519 N. Rosemead Blvd., Suite 101
Rosemead, CA 91770
626/285-2128, fax 626/285-2120
Adolescent and adult psychiatry; ADD in children.

Marijane Zimmerli, D.O.
716 Yarmouth Rd., Suite 203
Palos Verdes Estates, CA 90274
310/377-3070
Child, adolescent, and adult psychiatry.

ORANGE COUNTY AREA

The Amen Clinic Newport Beach
4019 Westerly Pl., Suite 100
Newport Beach, CA 92660
949/266-3700

Barton J. Blinder, M.D., Ph.D.
400 Newport Center Dr., #706
Newport Beach, CA 92660
949/640-4440, fax 949/721-9572
Adult, adolescent, and child psychiatry and psychoanalysis.

Willard Hawkins, M.D.
745 S. Brea Blvd., #21
Brea, CA 92921
714/256-2660, fax 714/256-0937
Family practice physician with interest in SPECT; ADHD management for
adults and children, mood disorders, assessments, and referral for SPECT.

William Rodman Shankle, M.D.
19782 MacArthur Blvd., #310
Irvine, CA 92612
949/833-2383, fax 949/838-0153
Neurology; specialist in dementia and related illnesses; see his website at
www.mccare.com.

Ted Williams, M.D.
1551 North Tustin Ave., Suite 540
Santa Ana, CA 92705-8634
714/835-6700, fax 714/835-4650
General psychiatry.

Joseph Wu, M.D.
UC Irvine, 163 Irvine Hall, Room 109 UC-BIC
Irvine, CA 92697
949/824-7867
Associate professor of psychiatry; clinical director of UC Irvine Brain Imaging Center at the college of medicine.

William Young, M.D.
17822 Beach Blvd., #437
Huntington Beach, CA 92647
714/842-9377
Child, adolescent, and adult psychiatry.

San Diego Area

Mark Kosins, M.D.
647 Camino de Los Mares, #200
San Clemente, CA 92673
949/489-9898, fax 949/489-2569
email: markkosins@aol.com
Psychiatry, all ages, psychopharmacology, assessments, referral for SPECT, psychotherapy, and counseling services.

Steven E. Rudolph, D.O.
3030 Children's Way, #101
San Diego, CA 92123-4208
858/966-6752, fax 858/966-6753
Child and adult psychiatry.

San Francisco Bay Area

The Amen Clinic Fairfield
350 Chadbourne Rd.
Fairfield, CA 94585
707/429-7181, fax 707/429-8219
Specializing in assessments, neuroimaging, medication management, psychotherapy, psychological testing for children, adolescents, and adults.

Samuel Benson, M.D.
590 Ygnacio Valley Rd., #302
Walnut Creek, CA 94596
925/938-8085, fax 925/935-8506

Timmen Cermak, M.D.
239 Miller Ave., Suite 1
Mill Valley, CA 94941
415/346-4460
Psychiatry.

Kirk Clopton, M.D.
1037 Suncast, #100
El Dorado Hills, CA 95762
916/939-2343
Child, adolescent, and adult psychiatry.

George Delgado, M.D., SAAFP
2012 Columbus Pkwy.
Benicia, CA 94510
707/745-2705
Board-certified in family practice with special interest in child and adult psychiatry, depression, ADHD, and Bipolar Disorder.

Rick Gilbert, M.D.
9051 Soquel Dr., Suite F
Aptos, CA 95003
408/688-6712
Psychiatry.

Richard Lavine, M.D.
271 Miller Ave.
Mill Valley, CA 94941
415/383-2882
Psychiatry.

Emmett Miller, M.D.
P.O. Box 803
Nevada City, CA 95959
530/478-1807

Psychotherapist specializing in ADD, deep relaxation, mind-body medicine, and hypnotherapy. Information on Dr. Miller's deep-relaxation and imagery tapes can be found at www.DrMiller.com.

Edward Oklan, M.D., MPH
Diplomat, American Board of Psychiatry and Neurology
811 San Anselmo Ave.
San Anselmo, CA 94960-2003
415/453-1797

Adult, adolescent, child psychiatry; expert in the use and interpretations of SPECT.

Hugh Ridlehuber, M.D.
1301 Ralston Ave., Suite C
Belmont, CA 94002
650/591-2345

Child, adolescent, and adult psychiatry.

C. Herbert Schiro, M.D.
47 Maria Dr., Suite 811 B
Yuba City, CA 95991
530/673-5331

Adult, adolescent, and child psychiatry.

Edward Spencer, M.D.
51 Marina Dr., Suite 821 B
Petaluma, CA 94954
707/763-6854

General neurology, SPECT brain imaging, epilepsy, dementia, migraine, ADHD.

Matthew Stubblefield, M.D.
3303 Alma St.
Palo Alto, CA 94306
650/856-0406
General child, adolescent, and adult psychiatrist; expert in ADHD and SPECT brain imaging.

George L. Wilkinson, M.D.
702 Marshall St., Suite 410
Redwood City, CA 94063
650/367-0472
Adult and forensic psychiatry; adult ADD.

Colorado

Daniel Hoffman, M.D.
8200 E. Belleview Ave., Suite 600E
Greenwood Village, CO 80111
303/741-4800
Neuropsychiatrist, neurofeedback, brain injuries, adults, and children.

Connecticut

Henry Mann, M.D.
188 Wolf Neck Rd.
Stonington, CT 06378
860/536-6023
Psychiatry.

District of Columbia

James Merikangas, M.D.
Georgetown University Hospital, Department of Psychiatry
Kober Cogan Building, Room 526
3800 Reservoir Rd., NW
Washington, D.C. 20007-2197
202/687-8609
Dr. Merikangas is director of the neuropsychiatry program and a neurologist and psychiatrist.

Florida

Thomas Moseley, M.D.
1351 Bedford Dr., Suite 103
Melbourne, FL 32940
321/757-6799
Child, adolescent, and adult psychiatrist.

Georgia

Joseph Berger, M.D.
1575 Northside Dr.
Atlanta, GA 30318
404/350-0001

2321 Henry Clower Blvd., Suite A
Snellville, GA 30078
770/978-6782
Psychiatrist.

Illinois

Steven Devore Best, M.D.
The Neuroscience Center
440 Lake Cook Rd., Suite 2
Deerfield, IL 60015
847/236-9310
Psychiatrist.

Georgia Davis, M.D.
1112 Rickard Rd., Suite B
Springfield, IL 62704
217/787-9540
Child, adolescent, and adult psychiatry.

Phillip Epstein, M.D.
800/200-6564
Psychiatrist.

Richard L Grant, M.D.
709 Townes Ct.
Peoria, IL 61615
309/692-5550
Psychiatrist.

Robert Kohn, D.O.
5404 W. Elm St. Place # Q
McHenry, IL 60050
815/344-7951
www.brain-spect.com
Brain SPECT; practice limited to neurology and psychiatry; assistant clinical professor of radiology, University of Illinois, Chicago.

Dan G. Pavel, M.D. (referral for programming SPECT studies)
Professor of Radiology/Nuclear Medicine
Assistant Department Head for Information Systems
Department of Radiology
University of Illinois Medical Center at Chicago
Chicago, IL 60612
312/996-3961

Ivan A. Wolfson, Psy.D.
649 Ridgeview Dr.
McHenry, IL 60050
630/539-4987
Licensed clinical psychologist

Minnesota

A.W. Atkinson, M.D.
Associates 2000, PA
206 S. Broadway, Suite 601
Rochester, MN 55904
507/282-1009, fax 507/282-0932
www.associates2000pa.com
Board-certified in pediatrics; board certified, developmental-behavioral pediatrics.

Susan C. Jenkins, M.D.
Associates 2000, PA, Medical Director
206 S. Broadway, Suite 601
Rochester, MN 55904
507/282-1009, fax 507/282-0932
www.associates2000pa.com
Board-certified in child, adolescent, and adult psychiatry.

Nebraska

Thomas Jaeger, M.D.
2430 S. 73rd St., Suite 201
Omaha, NE 68124
402/392-2205
Child and adolescent psychiatrist.

Nevada

Corydon Clark, M.D.
2373-A Renaissance Dr.
Las Vegas, NV 89119
702/736-1919
Child, adolescent, and adult psychiatry, ADD, OCD, Tourette's, mood and anxiety disorders; Bipolar and Asperger's disorder.

Pennsylvania

Howard Baker, M.D.
1421 Walnut St., Suite 1412
Philadelphia, PA 19102
215/735-7141
Specialty: ADHD evaluations; treatment (adults and adolescents); medication management.

Margaret Baker, Ph.D.
1200 Remington Rd.
Wynnewood, PA 19096-2330
610/896-9651
Specialty: ADHD evaluations; psychological testing and psychotherapeutic treatment of ADHD in adults, adolescents, and children.

Joseph Kosakoski, M.D.
230 Harrisburg Ave., Suite 8
Lancaster, PA 17603
717/509-1931 or 717/509-1933
Psychiatry.

Tennessee

Robert Hunt, M.D.
2129 Belcourt Ave.
Nashville, TN 37212
615/383-1222
Child, adolescent, and adult psychiatry/SPECT imaging.

Texas

Lisa C. Routh, M.D.
7505 Fannin Road, Suite 510
Houston, TX 77054
713/790-0754, fax 713/790-1302
State-of-the-art brain SPECT imaging facility located in the Texas Medical
Center. Dynamic staff and innovative practice design. Adult, child, and adolescent psychiatry; hormonal and chemical imbalance; traumatic brain injury.

Utah

Susan Mirow, Ph.D., M.D.
Dept. of Psychiatry, University of Utah
Salt Lake City, UT 84132
801/532-1212, fax 801/532-1333
Psychiatry.

Washington

Clark T. Ballard, Jr., M.D.
1715 114th Ave., SE, Suite 208
Bellevue, WA 98004
425/452-0700, fax 425/450-6674
Psychiatry.

Theodore Mandelkorn, M.D., and Janice Woolley, M.D.
2553 76th Ave., SE
Mercer Island, WA 98040-2758
206/275-0702
Behavioral pediatrics.

Terrance McGuire, M.D.
1715 114th Ave., SE, #208
Bellevue, WA 98004
425/452-0700

618 NE Harrison St.
Poulsbo, WA 98370
425/452-0700
General psychiatry, ADD specialty.

Robert Sands, M.D.
The Amen Clinic Northwest
3315 South 23rd, Suite 100
Tacoma, WA 98405
253/779-HOPE (4673)
Psychiatry.

Therapists

Alaska

Linda Webber, Ph.D., and Leon Webber, DMn, LMFT
135 Christensen Dr., Suite 100
Anchorage, AK 99501
907/276-4910
Individual and family therapists; specialty in couples, ADD, and related
disorders.

California

Charles Ara, Ph.D., MFCC
11215 Park St.

Cerritos, CA 90703
562/865-4075

Kim Barrus, Ph.D., FPPR
Clinical psychologist
2239 Townsgate Rd., Suite 107
Westlake Village, CA 91361
818/597-0292, fax 401/679-8644
ADD, depression, and anxiety; works with Amen Clinic principles.

Sheila Bastien, Ph.D.
2126 Los Angeles Ave.
Berkeley, CA 94707
510/526-7391
Neuropsychologist.

Susan Brown, LCSW
Lifeforce Services, Inc.
4700 Spring St., #204
La Mesa, CA 91941
619/698-5435
Specializes in EMDR.

Jamie Baudizzon, LCSW
1933 Market St., Suite C
Redding, CA 96001
530/241-9276, fax 530/241-0114
Addictions; criminal justice specialist; therapy; special master cases for the court, custody issues.

Sara G. Gilman, MFT
Lifeforce Services, Inc.
374 North Coast Hwy 101, Suite F-15
Encinitas, CA 92024
www.lifeforceservices.com
760/942-8663
Specializes in EMDR, PTSD, depression.

Dennis Gowans, Ph.D.
14603 E. Whittier Blvd.
Whittier, CA 90605
562/945-6471

Jan Hackelman, R.N.
1090 E. Washington St., Suite B
Colton, CA 92324
909/730-6575

Earl Henslin, Psy.D.
745 S. Brea, Suite 23
Brea, CA 92821
714/256-4673, fax 714/256-0937
Large group practice with adult and child therapists; SPECT referrals, assessments, and therapy. Dr. Henslin is a published author and a highly sought-after public speaker.

Corrine Hickson, Ph.D.
25550 Hawthorne Blvd., Suite 212
Torrance, CA 90503
310/810-0349; 310/375-8665
HicksonSI@aol.com

Gabriele Hillberg, Ph.D.
1669 Gretel Ave.
Mountain View, CA 94040
650/314-0133

Connie Hornyak, LCSW
Attachment Center West
1538 Brookhollow Dr., Suite E
Santa Ana, CA 92705
714/751-7789, fax 714/751-7791
CHLCSW@PACBELL.NET
www.attachmentcenter.com

Lynn Jarvis, Ph.D., and David Jarvis, Ph.D.
3225 North Verdugo Rd.
Glendale, CA 91208
818/957-2060; 714/491-7832

Sheila Krystal, Ph.D.
1509 Euclid Ave.
Berkeley, CA 94708
510/540-0855
Transpersonal psychologist working with individuals and couples and specializing in ADD, anxiety and depression, and using cognitive therapy, EMDR, and meditation.

Mary Joann Lang, Ph.D.
901 Dove St., Suite 150
Newport Beach, CA 92660
949/752-6141
Neuropsychologist, testing in learning disabilities.

Karen Lansing, MFT, BCETS
3060 Valencia Ave., Suite 6
Aptos, CA 95003
831/460-2550
Marriage, family, and child counselor; specializes in treating law enforcement and emergency service personnel.

David Lechuga, Ph.D.
Neurobehavioral Clinic
27725 Santa Margarita Pkwy., Suite 221
Mission Viejo, CA 92691
949/837-3358, fax 949/837-0274
Neuropsychologist.

Jennifer Lendl, Ph.D.
Performance Enhancement Unlimited
1142 McKendrie St.
San Jose, CA 95126-1406
408/244-6186

Specializes in trauma and performance enhancement; EMDR trainer; has worked at the Amen Clinic Fairfield for many years.

Melvyn Lewin, Ph.D.
716 Yarmouth Rd.
Palos Verdes Estates, CA 90274
310/377-1198, fax 310/377-5827
Specializes in ADHD, difficult children, parent coaching, addiction.

Michael Linden, Ph.D.
30270 Rancho Viejo Rd., Suite C
San Juan Capistrano, CA 92675
800/ADD-9117
Specializes in neurofeedback, social skills groups, parent training, and psychotherapy.

Michael J. McGrath, MFCC
Psychological Services Building
825 De Long Ave.
Novato, CA 94945
415/899-1378
Specializing in working with adolescents and their families in addition to young adults.

Daniel McQuoid, Psy.D.
745 S. Brea Blvd., #23
Brea, CA 92821
714/256-4673

3545 Long Beach Blvd., #450
Long Beach, CA 90807
562/492-9162, ext. 5

Cynthia Nerio, MFT
CCCYL
5312 Richfield Rd.
Yorba Linda, CA 92886
714/562-6101, fax 714/777-1233

Linda Kozitza-Pepper, Ph.D.
Psychological Services
825 De Long Ave.
Novato, CA 94945
415/899-1379

Licensed psychologist in California and Oregon; specializes in the evaluation and treatment of children, adolescents, and adults with mood and attention disorders.

Marcel Ponton, Ph.D., QME
595 E. Colorado Blvd., Suite 800
Pasadena, CA 91101
800/314-7273, fax 800/307-9438

Specializes in brain injury.

Julia Ross, MA, Clinical Director
Recovery Systems
147 Lomita Dr., Suite D
Mill Valley, CA 94941
415/383-3611, x1
www.moodcure.com

Amino acid and other nutritional brain repair for mood problems, eating disorders, and addictions.

Saeed Soltani, Ph.D.
1551 N. Tustin Ave., #540
Santa Ana, CA 92705
714/835-1700

Specializes in compulsive disorders, ADD anxiety, Bipolar Disorder; substance abuse.

Veronika Tracy-Smith, Ph.D.
16052 Beach Blvd., Suite 228
Huntington Beach, CA 92647
714/841-3465

Specializes in neurofeedback, ADD, chronic pain, anxiety, depression, and migraines.

Turning Point Counseling Center
Kevin Downing, MFT
14943 Desman Rd.
La Mirada, CA 90635
www.turningpointcounseling.org
929/393-6366, ext. 8369
Intimacy in marriage; successful parenting; conflict and divorce prevention; men's issues; trauma recovery; attention deficit problems.

Heidi Yellen, MA, CET
Andrew Yellen, Ph.D.
11260 Wilbur Ave., Suite 303
Northridge, CA 91326
818/360-3078

Florida

Ray Bowman, Ph.D.
6740 Crosswood Dr. North
Saint Petersburg, FL 33710
727/345-1234

Scott Fairchild, Psy.D.
1351 Bedford Dr., Suite 103
Melbourne, FL 32940
321/757-6799

Idaho

Jonelle Sullivan Timlin, Ph.D.
302 N. 5th St.
Coeur d'Alene, ID 83814
208/664-3020, fax 208/664-3639
Specializes in child and adult psychology.

Illinois

John A. Atkin, LCSW
751 Roosevelt Rd., Suite 216
Glen Ellyn, IL 60137
630/545-2835
johnaatkin@yahoo.com
Specialty in working with adult and child ADD, depression, anxiety; cognitive behavioral therapy.

Ivan A. Wolfson, Psy.D.
Wolfson Psychological Services, LTD
Affiliated with The Kohn Group, LTD
32 E. Maple Ave.
Roselle, IL 60172-2246
630/539-4987

649 Ridgeview Dr.
McHenry, IL 60050
Specializing in individual and family treatment of ADHD and self-esteem-related difficulties, mood disorders; marital therapy.

Kansas

Linn Suderman, Ph.D.
2104 E W 25th St.
Lawrence, KS 66046
785/749-3838
Specialty in evaluating ADD and learning disabilities; transition in careers.

Louisiana

Craig Taffaro, Jr., MS, LPC
2118 Packenham Dr.
Chalmette, LA 70043
504/271-0546

Nevada

Tom Blitsch, MFT
1850 East Flamingo, Suite 137
Las Vegas, NV 89119
702/794-0317

Gregory Giron, Psy.D.
1201 Johnson St.
Carson City, NV 89706
775/885-4774
Behavioral health services, Division of Carson-Tahoe Clinic, ADHD clinic,
Adolescent Outpatient Services.

Ohio

Linda B. VanderPol-Lee, MA, MAHE, LPCC
3454 Oak Alley Court, Suite 410
Toledo, OH 43606
419/531-3337
lvanderp@buckeye-express.com

Oregon

Alec Mendelson, Ph.D.
1550 NW Eastman Pkwy., # 280
Gresham, OR 97030
503/665-4357, ext. 2
Child and adolescent psychologist; school-based psychological consultant.

Rory F. Richardson, Ph.D., FICPP
Clinical Psychologist and Neuropsychologist
4422 Devils Lake Rd., Suite 3
Lincoln City, OR 97367
541/994-4462
Specializing in assessment and treatment of children, adolescents, and adults
with complicated disorders including Bipolar Disorder, OCD, ADHD, neu-
rologic dysfunction, and others.

Texas

Elise Orman, Ph.D.
4608 South Lamar Blvd.
Austin, TX 78745
512/892-9355

Washington

Diane E. Hough, MS, LMHC, NCC
9725 SE 36th St., # 212
Mercer Island, WA 98040
206/275-4176, fax 425/369-8694

Specializing in child, adolescent, and adult therapy including consultation on parenting, child development, academic success, marriage, and coaching. She is a frequent trainer and presenter and specialist in SPECT applications and diagnosis for mood disorders and attention issues.

Kathy Marshack, Ph.D.
14237 SE Evergreen Hwy.
Vancouver, WA 98683
360/256-0448
www.kmarshack.com

4700 Macadam
Portland, OR 97201
503/222-6678

Therapist who understands SPECT very well; good resource for helping people locate doctor.

Diana Tognazzini, Ph.D.
6212 75th St. W.
Lakewood, WA 98499
253/589-8603

Clinical psychologist/school psychologist specializing in cognitive testing and adolescent school issues.

Amen/Routh
Anxiety/Depression
Algorithm

Our algorithm is designed as a quick reference and summary guide to the diagnostic and treatment principles for the seven types of anxiety and depression. Individual treatment plans may deviate from this general flowsheet.

A/D Type	Type 1 Pure Anxiety	Type 2 Pure Depression	Type 3 Mixed A&D
Symptom Clusters	Anxiety, nervousness, driven, panic attacks, fearful, self-doubt, avoidant behaviors, muscle tension, nail biting, headaches, abdominal pain, heart palpitations, shortness of breath, irrational fears/phobias, predicts the worst, startles easily	Persistent sad/negative mood; loss of interest in usually fun activities; periods of crying; frequent feelings of guilt, helplessness, hopelessness, or worthlessness; sleep and appetite changes (too much or too little); low energy levels; suicidal thoughts or attempts; pessimism	Combination of both Pure Anxiety symptoms and Pure Depression symptoms; one type may predominate at any point in time, but both symptom clusters are present on a regular basis
Traditional Diagnostic Categories (DSM-IV)	Generalized Anxiety Disorder, Panic Disorder, Agoraphobia	Major Depressive Episode, Dysthymia	Depression complicated by anxiety disorders vs. anxiety disorder complicated by depression; also, atypical depressions and depressions complicated by chronic pain
Typical SPECT Findings	Basal ganglia hyperactivity	Deep limbic hyperactivity at rest and during concentration, and decreased prefrontal cortex activity at rest that improves with concentration	Mixture of basal ganglia and deep limbic hyperactivity

Type 4 Overfocused	Type 5 Cyclic	Type 6 Temporal Lobe	Type 7 Unfocused A&D
Trouble shifting attention, gets stuck on negative thoughts or behaviors, worries, upset when things are out of place, dislikes change, needs to have things done a certain way, holds grudges, oppositional or argumentative, tends to start answers with "no" more common in children or grandchildren of alcoholics	Cyclic moods are the hallmark; periods of elevated, depressed, or anxious moods; periods of altered sleep and appetite; thoughts may race; periods of markedly increased or decreased energy levels; periods of poor judgment	Temper outbursts; memory problems; mood instability; visual or auditory illusions, and dark, suicidal, frightening or evil thoughts; misinterprets comments in a negative way; trouble reading social situations; mild paranoia; may have episodes of panic or fear for no specific reason; frequent déjà vu; preoccupied with religious thoughts	Tired, low energy, trouble thinking and staying focused, spaciness, feeling overwhelmed, procrastination, failure to finish tasks, boredom, loses things, easily distracted, forgetful, poor planning skills, difficulty expressing feelings
Obsessive-Compulsive Disorder, Post-traumatic Stress Disorder, eating disorders, Tourette's syndrome, Obsessive-Compulsive Personality Disorder	Bipolar Disorder, Cyclothymia, recurrent depressions, Premenstrual Dysphoric Disorder (PMDD), Seasonal Affective Disorder (SAD)	Temporal Lobe Epilepsy, Borderline Personality Disorder	Attention Deficit Disorder with anxiety or depression
Anterior cingulate gyrus, basal ganglia, and/or deep limbic system hyperactivity	Focal increased activity in the deep limbic system and/or "ring of fire" or patchy increased activity	Increased or decreased activity in the temporal lobes with increased basal ganglia and/or deep limbic hyperactivity	Decreased activity in the prefrontal cortex and increased activity in the basal ganglia and/or deep limbic system

(continued)

A/D Type	Type 1 Pure Anxiety	Type 2 Pure Depression	Type 3 Mixed A&D
Made Worse by	Stimulants	Stimulants	Stimulants
Diet	Higher protein, lower carbohydrate	Higher protein, lower carbohydrate	Higher protein, lower carbohydrate
Exercise	Intense aerobic	Intense aerobic	Intense aerobic
Herbs, Supplements	GABA, kava, L-glutamine, valerian	DL-phenylalanine, L-tyrosine, SAMe	Combination of type 1 and 2 supplements
Medications	Buspar, limited use of benzodiaze-pines, anticon-vulsants	Buproprion, desipramine, imipramine	Imipramine, or combinations of Type 1 and 2 supplements
Psychosocial Treatments	Biofeedback, ANT therapy, relaxa-tion, meditation	ANT therapy, interpersonal psychotherapy	Biofeedback, ANT therapy, inter-personal psycho-therapy, relaxation, meditation

Type 4 Overfocused	Type 5 Cyclic	Type 6 Temporal Lobe	Type 7 Unfocused A&D
Stimulants	All antidepressants, including supplement SAMe, can trigger a manic episode in vulnerable people	Selective serotonin reuptake inhibitors, stimulants, or stimulating antidepressants, such as Wellbutrin, supplements that increase serotonin levels	Selective serotonin reuptake inhibitors, sedatives
Lower protein, higher carbohydrate	Higher protein, lower carbohydrate	Higher protein, lower carbohydrate	Higher protein, lower carbohydrate
Intense aerobic	Intense aerobic	Intense aerobic	Intense aerobic
St. John's wort, 5-HTP, L-tyrptophan, Inositol	GABA, taurine, fish oil, gingko biloba, phosphytidal serine, vitamin E, Piracetam	GABA, taurine, fish oil, gingko biloba, phosphytidal serine, vitamin E, Piracetam	L-tyrosine, DL-phenylalanine, SAMe
Serotonin-enhancing meds such as Effexor, Zoloft, Paxil, Prozac, Celexa, or Luvox; novel antipsychotics for severe cases	Anticonvulsants such as Depakote, Carbatrol, Neurontin, Topamax, Lamictal, Gabatril, Dilantin	Anticonvulsants such as Depakote, Carbatrol, Neurontin, Topamax, Lamictal, Gabatril, Dilantin	Stimulants or stimulating antidepressants
Distraction, ANT therapy, relaxation, meditation	Stress reduction, interpersonal psychotherapy	Supportive psychotherapy	Dance, stimulating music

CHAPTER 20

32 Strategies to Overcome Anxiety and Depression

1. Get help early.

2. Become a master at diaphragmatic (belly) breathing.

3. Do not believe every thought or feeling you have. Thoughts and feelings are based on complex memories and chemical reactions; sometimes they lie to you.

4. Become a master ANTeater; watch out for the ANTs (automatic negative thoughts) that ruin your mood.

5. Exercise (sweat and get your heart rate up) four to five times a week.

6. Diet matters . . . for your type. Plan your meals.

7. Meditate to calm the emotional centers of your brain and to encourage a more relaxed, happy state.

8. If you want to avoid or lessen the amount of medication for anxiety and depression, use meditation, physical exercise, proper nutrition, and the ANT-eating techniques outlined in the book.

9. Healing relationships enhances mood and calms anxiety. Continue to build positive relationships in your life—practice clear communication, cooperation, and forgiveness.

10. Find the best professional/specialist you can. Take your time, get second or third opinions, and go outside your insurance plan if necessary. The initial investment in an excellent treatment plan saves far

more money in the long run than cutting corners on health care by staying with HMOs and PPOs.

11. If several medications are needed, first choose medication to deal with the most significant symptoms.

12. Start one medication at a time and make only one medication change at follow-up visits.

13. Do not be afraid to use combination medications (29 percent of the U.S. population have two separate problems, 17 percent have three).

14. Patients with severe symptoms may need three or even four medications together (typically an anticonvulsant, stimulant, and antidepressant).

15. When there are both temporal lobe and anterior cingulate gyrus (overfocus) problems, treat the temporal lobe issues first.

16. Less is not better. Strive for the best dose, not the least amount possible.

17. Medication by itself is not the best treatment for anxiety and/or depression. Bio-psycho-social treatment is best with a combination of education, support, medicine or supplements, diet, exercise, and targeted psychotherapeutic techniques.

18. Keep a daily mood log to monitor progress.

19. Have your spouse or parents go to some doctor appointments with you if they are having trouble understanding your condition or your need to take medication. Also, having someone who knows you well go to an appointment with you can give your doctor background information that may be helpful.

20. Be an advocate for your own treatment. If you're confused about your diagnosis or if you aren't getting better, ask your doctor about further tests and SPECT scans to evaluate your brain function. This will help with diagnosis and treatment planning.

21. Understand brain system functions and problems so you know what treatments are likely to be most effective for you personally.

22. Consider alternative interventions for mild to moderate conditions but remember that conventional medications are usually required for moderate to severe problems.

23. Suicide is a permanent solution to a temporary feeling or problem. Things often look better in the morning. Get help through a hotline, a counselor, or your physician.

24. Adopt a healthy lifestyle by starting small. Start by cutting back or eliminating caffeine and nicotine (they constrict blood flow to the brain). You might get a brief boost in the short run, but these are bad actors over time.

25. Anxiety and depression runs in families. If one person has it, it is often helpful to screen others for it.

26. Education helps to decrease the impact an anxious and depressed person has on family members. Anxiety and depression affects everyone in the family. Having family members attend appointments and join support groups and read literature are ways of educating them about anxiety and depression.

27. Practice our techniques for getting a good night's sleep. Sleep is essential. Use good sleep hygiene to get between six and nine hours a night.

28. Come prepared to doctor visits, with written questions and concerns. Talk about positive effects, side effects, and what other help you need.

29. Talk to your doctor about sexual side effects of medications. There are many things that can be done to try to counteract them.

30. Make no excuses to avoid treatment. There are safe protocols for children, pregnant and nursing women, medically fragile people, and the elderly.

31. Honesty is the best policy. Tell your doctor about every supplement, vitamin, herb, and other medication you take. Don't minimize the amount of nicotine or caffeine that you use, and no matter what your concerns are, never, ever hold back information about illegal drug use. If you have concerns about what your doctor will do with the information or who might see it, by all means ask those questions, but don't ever withhold the information. Your life might depend on drug interactions.

32. When treatment doesn't work, be persistent; with continued advances in medicine we are able to help more and more people.

RECOMMENDED READING

EDUCATION IS ESSENTIAL for a full understanding of your disorder and your issues. You may find the following books very helpful:

The Bipolar Child: The Definitive and Reassuring Guide to Childhood's Most Misunderstood Disorder, Demitri Papolos, M.D., and Janice Papolos. Broadway Books, revised and expanded edition, 416 pages, 2002.

Bipolar Disorders: A Guide to Helping Children and Adolescents, Mitzi Waltz. Patient-Centered Guides, 442 pages, 2000.

Body for Life, Bill Phillips and Michael D'Orso (contributor). HarperCollins, 224 pages, 1999.

Change Your Brain, Change Your Life, Daniel G. Amen, M.D. Times Books, 337 pages, 2000.

Coaching Yourself to Success, Daniel G. Amen, M.D. Mindworks Press, 339 pages, 1994.

The Diet Cure: The 8-Step Program to Rebalance Your Body Chemistry and End Food Cravings, Weight Problems, and Mood Swings—Now, Julia Ross. Penguin USA, 416 pages, reissue 2000.

Driven to Distraction: Recognizing and Coping with Attention Deficit Disorder from Childhood Through Adulthood, Edward M. Hallowell and John J. Ratey. Touchstone Books, 319 pages, 1995.

The Feeling Good Handbook, David Burns, M.D. Plume, 729 pages, 1999.

Healing ADD: The Breakthrough Program That Allows You to See and Heal the 6 Types of ADD, Daniel G. Amen, M.D. Berkley Publishing Group, 448 pages, 2002.

Healing the Greatest Hurt, Matthew Linn, et al. Paulist Press, 244 pages, 1985.

The Mayo Clinic Williams-Sonoma Cookbook: Simple Solutions for Eating Well, The Mayo Clinic, et al. Time Life, 272 pages, 1998.

Mind Over Mood, Dennis Greenberger and Christine A. Padesky. Guilford Press, 243 pages, 1995.

The Mood Cure: The 4-Step Program to Rebalance Your Emotional Chemistry and Rediscover Your Natural Sense of Well-Being, Julia Ross. Viking Press, 352 pages, 2002.

The Mozart Effect: Tapping the Power of Music to Heal the Body, Strengthen the Mind, and Unlock the Creative Spirit, Don Campbell. Avon Books, 332 pages, 1997.

New Hope for People with Bipolar Disorder, Jan Fawcet, M.D., et al. Prima Publishing, 352 pages, 2000.

The Promise of Sleep, William Dement, M.D. AudioBook, Amazon.com.

Protein Power: The High Protein/Low Carbohydrate Way to Lose Weight, Feel Fit, and Boost Your Health—in Just Weeks, Michael R. Eades, M.D., and Mary Dan Eades, M.D. Bantam Books, 429 pages, 1997.

The Relaxation and Stress Reduction Workbook, Martha Davis, et al., fifth edition. New Harbinger Publications, 276 pages, 2000.

Straight Talk About Psychiatric Medications for Kids, Timothy E. Wilens. Guilford Press, 279 pages, 1998.

Taking Charge of ADHD, revised edition, Russell A. Barkley. Guilford Press, 321 pages, 2000.

Wherever You Go, There You Are: Mindful Meditation in Everyday Life, Jon Kabat-Zinn. Hyperion, 278 pages, 1995.

The Zone: A Dietary Road Map to Lose Weight Permanently: Reset Your Genetic Code: Prevent Disease: Achieve Maximum Physical Performance, Barry Sears and Bill Lawren. HarperCollins, 352 pages, 1995.

INTERNET RESOURCES

www.adaa.org—Anxiety Disorders Association of America

www.ADD.org This is an outstanding website of the National ADD Association that contains advice, a listing of support groups, and research updates.

www.algy.com/anxiety. The Anxiety Panic Internet Resource sponsors this excellent self-help resource for people with anxiety disorders. Information on OCD, panic disorder, and PTSD.

www.Bipolarawareness.com. Information on Bipolar Disorder, how to talk to a physician, rating scales.

www.Lilly.com. Sponsored by Eli Lilly and Co., patients can access information about drugs such as Zyprexa, Prozac, and others.

www.consumerlab.com. Excellent, user-friendly website that allows people to access information necessary to evaluate vitamins, supplements, herbal preparations, and medication for purity, ease of absorption, and so forth.

www.Concerta.net, by the Concerta Center of Attention Program. Information for patients and families about ADHD, treatment, and Concerta.

www.ncptsd.org, by the National Center for PTSD. Website contains concise articles about the diagnosis and treatment of PTSD, current research, frequently asked questions, and assessment instruments.

www.healthybeginning.com. Highly animated site designed to assist adults in helping children to develop healthy habits at an early age. Includes guides for families and teachers.

www.nih.gov/health/consumer/conicd.htm. Fact sheets, information, and educational brochures about a host of topics including anxiety, aging, and depression from the National Institutes of Health.

www.MayoClinic.com. Award-winning website with information about mental health, nutrition, medications, and links to other sites.

www.psychiatry24x7.com. Available round-the-clock resources for psychiatry, mood calendars, and checklists.

www.safemedication.com—American Society of Health-System Pharmacists. Type in the name of medications to access information about drugs, when and how to take them, and alternative medication (when it may or may not be appropriate).

www.foodfit.com. One hundred award-winning professional chefs contribute great healthy recipes to this site. Also cooking and fitness advice.

www.ocfoundation.org—Obsessive Compulsive (OC) Foundation

www.psych.org—American Psychiatric Association

www.apa.org—American Psychological Association

www.aabt.org—Association for Advancement of Behavior Therapy

www.nmha.org—National Mental Health Association

www.ncptsd.org—National Center for PTSD

www.ndmda.org—National Depressive and Manic Depressive Association. An excellent educational and advocacy organization.

www.support-group.com. Support-Group.com—a collection of electronic support group links including depression.

www.pendulum.org—Pendulum resources—a page with information and links regarding Bipolar Disorder.

www.aacap.org—American Academy of Child-Adolescent Psychiatry—great for parents.

www.psycom.net/depression.central.html—Depression Central—the homepage by Dr. Ivan Goldberg; full of useful information and resources on depression.

www.mentalhealth.com—Internet Mental Health—a great source of information.

www.nami.org—National Alliance for the Mentally Ill (NAMI)—terrific organization working to help the mentally ill.

www.bipolarchild.com—The Bipolar Child website.

ACKNOWLEDGMENTS

WE ARE GRATEFUL to the best teachers that physicians can have—our patients. We wish to acknowledge and thank the staff of the Amen Clinics, especially through all of the growing pains over the past fourteen years. We wish to thank both the professional staff and the support staff of the Amen Clinics.

We are grateful to have an amazing literary team. Our literary agent Faith Hamlin is the very best. She continually pushes us to be effective communicators, and she is a constant source of wisdom, friendship, and support. Thanks to our editor at Putnam, Sheila Oakes, and our wonderful publicist Tammy Richards, who has believed in and supported us through this book, as well as three others, by Dr. Amen.

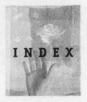

INDEX

Page numbers in italics refer to illustrations.

ABOUT THE AUTHORS

DANIEL G. AMEN, M.D., is a clinical neuroscientist, psychiatrist, and director of the Amen Clinics in Newport Beach and Fairfield, California, as well as in Tacoma, Washington. He is a nationally recognized expert in the field of "the brain and behavior," and lectures to thousands of psychiatrists, neurologists, psychologists, psychotherapists, and judges each year. Dr. Amen has pioneered the clinical use of brain SPECT imaging in psychiatry. The Amen Clinics have the world's largest database of brain images relating to behavior. He has presented his groundbreaking research on brain imaging and behavior internationally.

Dr. Amen did his psychiatric training at the Walter Reed Army Medical Center in Washington, D.C. He has won writing and research awards from the American Psychiatric Association, the U.S. Army, and the Baltimore-D.C. Institute for Psychoanalysis. Dr. Amen has been published around the world. He is the author of numerous professional and popular articles and nineteen books, including *Change Your Brain, Change Your Life*; *Healing ADD*; and *Healing the Hardware of the Soul*.

LISA C. ROUTH, M.D., is a neuropsychiatrist with special training in neurology, general psychiatry, child psychiatry, and functional brain imaging. She is a graduate of Texas A&M University College of Medicine and received specialty training at the Mayo Clinic in Rochester, Minnesota, and Timberlawn Hospital in Dallas, Texas. Dr. Roth is licensed in nuclear brain imaging and was formerly the medical director of the Amen Clinic in Newport Beach. She is currently at the University of Texas Medical Branch, Galveston, Texas. Dr. Routh is the mother of five, including two sets of twins, and is Native American. She has extensive experience with traumatic brain injury, disabled children, gender issues, and cross-cultural issues. Dr. Routh has diagnosed and treated thousands of people with depression and anxiety. She is a gifted teacher and speaks nationally on psychopharmacology, women's issues, and anxiety and depression.

The Amen Clinics

THE AMEN CLINICS were established in 1989 by Daniel G. Amen, M.D. They specialize in innovative diagnosis and treatment planning for a wide variety of behavioral, learning, and emotional problems for children, teenagers, and adults. The clinics have an international reputation for evaluating brain-behavior problems, such as Attention Deficit Disorder (ADD), depression, anxiety, school failure, brain trauma, Obsessive-Compulsive Disorders, aggressiveness, cognitive decline, and brain toxicity from drugs or alcohol. Brain SPECT imaging is performed in the clinics. The Amen Clinics have the world's largest database of brain scans for behavioral problems in the world. Over the last twelve years, they have performed more than 17,000 brain SPECT studies.

The clinics welcome referrals from physicians, psychologists, social workers, marriage and family therapists, drug and alcohol counselors, and individual clients.

The Amen Clinic Newport Beach
4019 Westerly Pl., Suite 100
Newport Beach, CA 92660
949/266-3700

The Amen Clinic Fairfield
350 Chadbourne Rd.
Fairfield, CA 94585
707/429-7181

The Amen Clinic Northwest
3315 South 23rd, Suite 100
Tacoma, WA 98405
253/779-HOPE (4673)
www.amenclinic.com

Brainplace.com

Brainplace.com is an educational interactive brain website geared toward mental health and medical professionals, educators, students, and the general public. It contains a wealth of information to help you learn about the brain. The site contains more than 300 color brain SPECT images, hundreds of scientific abstracts on brain SPECT imaging for psychiatry, a brain puzzle, an eighteen-minute video on brain SPECT imaging, and much, much more.

View more than 300 astonishing color 3D brain SPECT images on:

Aggression

Anxiety disorders

Attention Deficit Disorder, including the six subtypes

Brain trauma

Dementia and cognitive decline

Depression

Drug abuse

Obsessive-Compulsive Disorder

PMS

Seizures

Stroke